Osteonecrosis
of the Femoral Head

Rafael J. Sierra
Editor

Osteonecrosis
of the Femoral Head

A Clinical Casebook

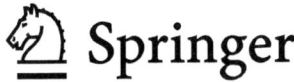 Springer

Editor
Rafael J. Sierra
Mayo Clinic
Rochester, Minnesota, USA

ISBN 978-3-319-50662-3   ISBN 978-3-319-50664-7   (eBook)
DOI 10.1007/978-3-319-50664-7

Library of Congress Control Number: 2017936710

Printed on acid-free paper

This Springer imprint is published by Springer Nature
The registered company is Springer International Publishing AG
The registered company address is: Gewerbestrasse 11, 6330 Cham, Switzerland

Preface

This first edition of *Osteonecrosis of the Femoral Head: A Clinical Casebook* assembles the various treatment options available for management of osteonecrosis of the femoral head (ONFH). Its goal is to provide the practicing hip surgeon and medical practitioner with an easy-to-read, case-based discussion on the modern treatment of ONFH, with special emphasis on early or pre-collapse stages.

The prevalence of ONFH seems to be on the rise and related to the medical treatment of life-threatening conditions such as cancers, organ transplantation, and/or treatment of rheumatologic conditions with a combination of steroid regimens. The condition affects very young patients and unfortunately still carries a fairly poor prognosis if left untreated. Diagnosing the condition early will give us the option of treating this condition in early stages in order to delay or avoid completely total hip arthroplasty (THA). Although THA is an option for late-stage ON, it is imperative for us to understand the pros and cons of the various surgical procedures that have been performed around the world for the management of early-stage ON in an effort to provide pain relief and delay progression. This book compiles a number of treatment options for management of early-stage ON. Furthermore, the treatment of post-collapse ON is discussed, presenting cases of several salvage procedures or THA.

We gathered leaders from around the world to discuss the surgical treatment for this condition and their outcomes. In each chapter, a description of the patient, the work-up and diagnosis, and surgical strategies are presented, with an in-depth discussion of the potential pitfalls or complications that can occur with each procedure. The reader will therefore obtain the knowledge required for managing the patient and understand the surgical technique and complexity of the procedure to be performed.

The innovative format of this book represents the future of medical education. More and more conferences are moving toward case-based format education as it represents for the clinician a real-life situation that is easy to remember and learn. This is the first book to gather the combined international experience for treatment of ON, uniting treatment recommendations across three continents. I have to thank the chapter authors for their expertise, for their lifelong journey in studying and treating this difficult condition, and certainly for dedicating the time that was required to write the chapters. I would like to acknowledge the support and assistance of Springer and their contributors for the organization of the chapters and dedicate this book to my wife, Victoria, and my two children, Sofia and Rafico, for their continued support throughout the years.

Rochester, MN, USA   Rafael J. Sierra

Contents

Contributors

C. Lowry Barnes, MD Department of Orthopaedic Surgery, University of Arkansas for Medical Sciences, Little Rock, AR, USA

Jeffrey J. Cherian, DO Center for Joint Preservation and Replacement, Rubin Institute for Advanced Orthopaedics, Sinai Hospital of Baltimore, Baltimore, MD, USA

Michele D'Apuzzo, MD The Center for Advanced Orthopaedics at Larkin, South Miami, FL, USA

Arnaud Dubory, MD Department of Orthopaedic Surgery, University Paris East, Créteil, France

Paul K. Edwards, MD Department of Orthopaedic Surgery, University of Arkansas for Medical Sciences, Little Rock, AR, USA

Randa K. Elmallah, MD Center for Joint Preservation and Replacement, Rubin Institute for Advanced Orthopaedics, Sinai Hospital of Baltimore, Baltimore, MD, USA

Richard A. Freiberg, MD Cholesterol, Metabolism, and Thrombosis Center, Jewish Hospital of Cincinnati and from the Division of Orthopaedics', VA Hospital, Cincinnati, OH, USA

Charles J. Glueck, MD Cholesterol, Metabolism, and Thrombosis Center, Jewish Hospital of Cincinnati and from the Division of Orthopaedics', VA Hospital, Cincinnati, OH, USA

Eric M. Greber, MD Department of Orthopaedic Surgery, University of Arkansas for Medical Sciences, Little Rock, AR, USA

Philippe Hernigou, MD Department of Orthopaedic Surgery, University Paris East, Créteil, France

Matthew T. Houdek, MD Department of Orthopaedic Surgery, Mayo Clinic, Rochester, MN, USA

Julio J. Jauregui, MD Center for Joint Preservation and Replacement, Rubin Institute for Advanced Orthopaedics, Sinai Hospital of Baltimore, Baltimore, MD, USA

Vasili Karas, MD Duke University Medical Center and Durham VA Medical Center, Durham, NC, USA

Stefan B. Keizer, MD Department of Orthopaedics, Haaglanden Medical Center, The Hague, The Netherlands

Charles Henri Flouzat Lachaniette, MD Department of Orthopaedic Surgery, University Paris East, Créteil, France

Carlos J. Lavernia, MD University of Miami, Florida International University, Coral Gables, FL, USA

Jay R. Lieberman, MD Department of Orthopaedic Surgery, Keck School of Medicine of USC, Los Angeles, CA, USA

J. Ryan Martin, MD OrthoCarolina, Matthews, NC, USA

Patrick Millikan, MD Duke University Medical Center and Durham VA Medical Center, Durham, NC, USA

Michael A. Mont, MD Center for Joint Preservation and Replacement, Rubin Institute for Advanced Orthopaedics, Sinai Hospital of Baltimore, Baltimore, MD, USA

Rob G.H.H. Nelissen, MD, PhD Department of Orthopaedics, Leiden University Medical Center, Leiden, The Netherlands

William C. Pannell, MD Department of Orthopaedic Surgery, Keck School of Medicine of USC, Los Angeles, CA, USA

Javad Parvizi, MD, FRCS James Edwards Professor of Orthopaedic Surgery, Sidney Kimmel School of Medicine, Rothman Institute at Thomas Jefferson University, Sheridan Building, Philadelphia, PA, USA

Todd P. Pierce, MD Center for Joint Preservation and Replacement, Rubin Institute for Advanced Orthopaedics, Sinai Hospital of Baltimore, Baltimore, MD, USA

Damien Potage, MD Department of Orthopaedic Surgery, University Paris East, Créteil, France

Rafael J. Sierra, MD Department of Orthopaedic Surgery, Mayo Clinic, Rochester, MN, USA

Robert T. Trousdale, MD Department of Orthopaedic Surgery, Mayo Clinic, Rochester, MN, USA

Hamed Vahedi, MD Rothman Institute at Thomas Jefferson University, Philadelphia, PA, USA

Jesus M. Villa, MD Arthritis Surgery Research Foundation, Coral Gables, FL, USA

Ping Wang, PhD Cholesterol, Metabolism, and Thrombosis Center, Jewish Hospital of Cincinnati and from the Division of Orthopaedics', VA Hospital, Cincinnati, OH, USA

Yisheng Wang, MD, PhD Department of Orthopaedic Surgery, 1st Affiliated Hospital of Zhengzhou University, Zhengzhou, Henan province, China

Samuel Wellman, MD Duke University Medical Center and Durham VA Medical Center, Durham, NC, USA

Cody C. Wyles, MD Department of Orthopaedic Surgery, Mayo Clinic, Rochester, MN, USA

Part I
Pre-collapse: Treatment of Early Stage Osteonecrosis

Chapter 1
Osteonecrosis and Thrombophilia: Pathophysiology, Diagnosis, and Treatment

Charles J. Glueck, Ping Wang, and Richard A. Freiberg

Case Presentation 1

This previously healthy 47-year-old female was started on an estrogen-testosterone patch to improve libido that was followed by the onset of intermittent right hip pain. When seen by us 2 years later, her pain had increased to the point that she could walk only short distances with a cane.

Diagnosis/Assessment

X-ray of the hips was normal, but MRI revealed Ficat stage I osteonecrosis of the right hip. There was no history of big-dose long-term steroids, alcoholism, or any other causes

C.J. Glueck, MD (✉) • P. Wang, PhD • R.A. Freiberg, MD
Cholesterol, Metabolism, and Thrombosis Center,
Jewish Hospital of Cincinnati and from the Division of
Orthopaedics', VA Hospital, Cincinnati, OH, USA
e-mail: cjglueck@mercy.com

R.J. Sierra (ed.), *Osteonecrosis of the Femoral Head*,
DOI 10.1007/978-3-319-50664-7_1,
© Mayo Foundation for Medical Education and Research 2017

for secondary osteonecrosis [1]. We carried out our usual diagnostic panel of laboratory tests of thrombophilia and hypofibrinolysis (Table 1.1). Studies of thrombophilia-hypofibrinolysis revealed previously undiagnosed heterozygosity for the prothrombin G20210A mutation, a thrombophilic, autosomal dominant mutation, associated with increased risk of venous thrombosis [2] and osteonecrosis [3]. All other coagulation tests, as displayed in Table 1.1, were negative. We believe that the osteonecrosis of the hip was caused by an interaction of the exogenous estrogen-testosterone and the thrombophilic prothrombin gene mutation [4].

Sonography of leg veins revealed no signs of deep venous thrombosis.

Management

The estrogen-testosterone patch was immediately discontinued. In the absence of contraindications to anticoagulation, enoxaparin 1.5 mg/kg/day in two divided doses was started. After completion of a 3-month course of enoxaparin, standard in our initial study protocol as required by the FDA [5], ambulation was pain-free. After being asymptomatic for an additional 8 months, right hip pain returned, and enoxaparin was restarted. After 3 months on the second course of enoxaparin, she again became asymptomatic. A repeat MRI revealed Ficat stage I osteonecrosis, without change from the pretreatment study.

Xarelto, 10 mg/day, was then started. She remained asymptomatic for the subsequent 9 months. Repeat MRI revealed no change, still Ficat stage I osteonecrosis.

Outcome

She remains entirely asymptomatic 3 years after initial diagnosis, being maintained on Xarelto 10 mg/day. In patients with major gene thrombophilias and Ficat stages I–II osteonecrosis at the time of first beginning anticoagulation, progression

TABLE 1.1 Coagulation disorders in patients with idiopathic and secondary osteonecrosis

	Factor V Leiden	PTG TC	PAIG 4G4G	MTHFR TT	Factor VIII >150%	Factor XI >150%	Homocysteine high[a]
Idiopathic osteonecrosis	20/220	10/213	59/210	44/211	39/161	10/154	24/196
(n = 221)	(9%)	(5%)	(28%)	(21%)	(24%)	(6%)	(12%)
Normal control	2/109	3/107	26/104	32/109	7/103	3/101	5/107
(n = 110)	(2%)	(3%)	(25%)	(29%)	(7%)	(3%)	(5%)
Idiopathic vs controls Fisher's p	.017	NS	NS	NS	.0002	NS	.04
Secondary osteonecrosis	9/111	3/109	31/109	32/110	10/69	3/61	17/108
(n = 113)	(8%)	(3%)	(28%)	(29%)	(14%)	(5%)	(16%)
Normal control	2/109	3/107	26/104	32/109	7/103	3/101	5/107
(n = 110)	(2%)	(3%)	(25%)	(29%)	(7%)	(3%)	(5%)
Secondary vs controls Fisher's p	.059	NS	NS	NS	NS	NS	.012

(continued)

TABLE 1.1 (continued)

	ACLA IgG high[b]	ACLA IgM high[c]	Antigenic Protein C <73%	Antigenic Protein S <63%	Antigenic Free S <66%	Antithrombin III <80%	Lupus positive
Idiopathic osteonecrosis	11/194	22/193	9/190	1/192	8/173	7/188	2/188
(n = 221)	(6%)	(11%)	(5%)	(0.5%)	(5%)	(4%)	(1%)
Normal control	6/109	2/109	6/96	4/96	2/96	2/96	2/110
(n = 110)	(6%)	(2%)	(6%)	(4%)	(2%)	(2%)	(2%)
Idiopathic vs controls Fisher's p	NS	.003	NS	.04	NS	NS	NS
Secondary osteonecrosis	5/106	10/106	3/100	3/99	16/95	2/97	5/101
(n = 113)	(5%)	(9%)	(3%)	(3%)	(17%)	(2%)	(5%)
Normal control	6/109	2/109	6/96	4/96	2/96	2/96	2/110

($n = 110$)	(6%)	(2%)	(6%)	(4%)	(2%)	(2%)	(2%)
Secondary vs controls Fisher's p	NS	.018	NS	NS	.0004	NS	NS

PTG prothrombin G20210A mutation, *PAIG* PAI-1 4G/5G promoter polymorphism, *MTHFR* methylenetetrahydrofolate reductase C677T/A1298C, *Free S* protein S free, *TT* homozygous mutant, *TC* heterozygote mutant, *CC* wild type normal

[a]Dated cut point for Homocysteine high: ≥13.5 *umol/l (before 3/20/2005); ≥12 (3/21/05–3/27/06); ≥10.4 (3/28/06–4/14/08); ≥11.4 (4/15/08–11/14/08); ≥15 (after 11/15/08)(6/9/15 revised)*

[b]Dated cut point for IgG high: ≥23 *GPL (before 10/31/12); ≥15 (after 11/1/12)*

[c]Dated cut point for IgM high: ≥10 *MPL (before 4/30/12); ≥13 (after 5/1/12)*

to joint collapse can usually be prevented, pain ameliorated, and function maintained [6]. Long-term anticoagulation also carries increased bleeding risk, but this is much less with the new Xa inhibitors than Coumadin [7–9].

Case Presentation 2

In January 2008, this 54-year-old Caucasian male developed increasing fatigue and loss of libido. Workup revealed low testosterone levels. A diagnosis of hypogonadism was made. He was then started on a testosterone patch (50 mg/ day) in February 2008. Six months after starting the testosterone patch, he developed severe bilateral hip pain. X-rays revealed bilateral osteonecrosis of the hips, right hip Ficat stage II and left Ficat stage I. On our evaluation of thrombophilia-hypofibrinolysis (Table 1.1), he was found to be heterozygous for the factor V Leiden mutation and homozygous for the MTHFR C677T mutation (associated with abnormal homocysteine metabolism). There were no risk factors for secondary osteonecrosis, and we attributed the development of the osteonecrosis to an interaction between the thrombophilic factor V Leiden mutation and exogenous testosterone therapy [4, 10].

Management

Testosterone was stopped. Enoxaparin, 1.5 mg/kg/day in two divided doses, was started and maintained for 3 months as usual. Four months later, MRI and X-ray showed no change from pretreatment, but his pain was much less. Because of persistent pain, a second 3-month course of enoxaparin was given, and he became asymptomatic. Eight months later, there was no change in his X-ray or MRI. Three years from initial treatment with enoxaparin, MRIs were unchanged. There were no new areas of osteonecrosis or marrow edema compared to pretreatment. Because of symptomatic improvement on enoxaparin and stable X-rays and magnetic resonance images (MRIs), chronic long-term anticoagulation was started 3 years after diagnosis with Pradaxa 150 mg twice per day.

Outcome

Five years after initial diagnosis, still on Pradaxa, no radiographic features of ON were identified in either hip. Nine years after diagnosis, still on Pradaxa, he remains asymptomatic, with no radiographic features of ON identified.

Case Presentation 3

This African-American female was originally seen at age 69 with severe left hip pain and moderately severe right hip pain. At pretreatment entry, X-rays revealed that the left hip was collapsed (Ficat stage III), but the right hip was Ficat II (Fig. 1.1). Coagulation tests

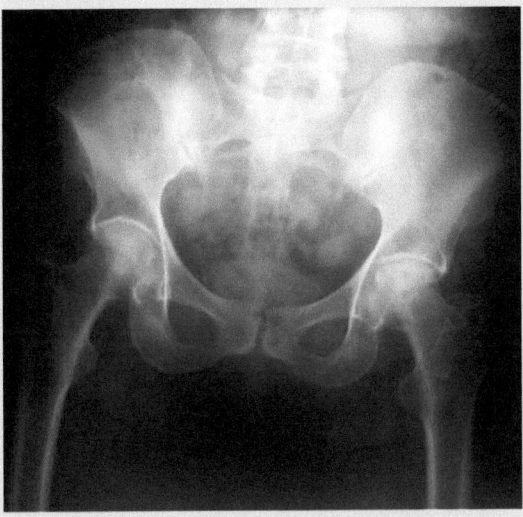

FIGURE I.I Pretreatment hip X-ray, Case #3. *Left* hip collapsed (Ficat stage (III), *right* hip Ficat stage II

revealed resistance to activated protein C, but PCR revealed wild-type normal factor V without the Leiden mutation. In such cases, there is usually a different mutation in the factor V gene (factor V Cambridge) [11], but the clinical thrombophilia is the same as if there were factor V Leiden heterozygosity.

Management

Because of financial constraints, anticoagulation was started with Coumadin rather than the usual enoxaparin. After 16 months on Coumadin, the right hip was asymptomatic and was unchanged on X-ray examination (Fig. 1.2). Total hip replacement was done on the left, as expected with Ficat III classification at presentation. In all of our studies

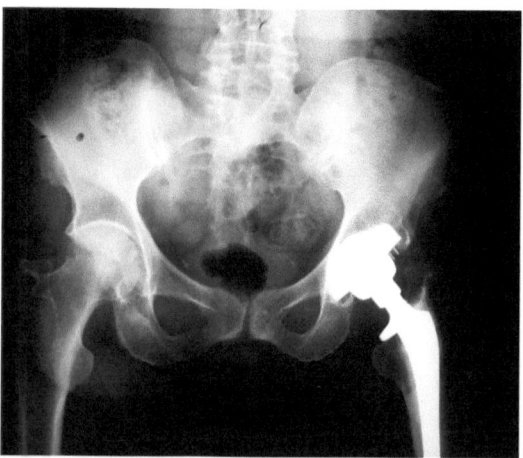

FIGURE 1.2 Hip X-ray after 16 months on Coumadin. *Right* hip Ficat stage II, unchanged from pretreatment. Total hip replacement had been done on the Ficat stage III *left* hip

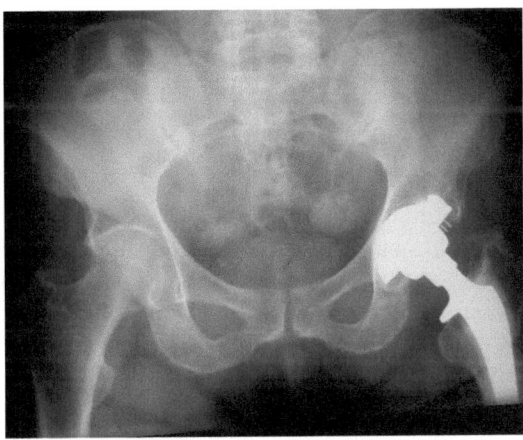

FIGURE 1.3 Hip X-ray after 13 years on Coumadin. *Right* hip Ficat stage II, unchanged from pretreatment

of anticoagulation in patients with idiopathic osteonecrosis with one hip or knee Ficat stage I or II compared to patients with stage III or IV, almost all the Ficat stage I–II joints were protected by anticoagulant treatment and did not manifest progression, but the stage III–IV joints progressed despite anticoagulation, usually requiring total joint replacement [5, 6, 12, 13]. After 13 years on Coumadin, the right hip remained asymptomatic, and the X-ray was unchanged (Ficat stage II) (Fig. 1.3).

Outcome

Within 16 months on Coumadin, the right hip became symptom-free and remained symptom-free for 11.5 subsequent years, for a total of 13 years on anticoagulation. In patients whose idiopathic Ficat stages I or II osteonecrosis are associated with familial thrombophilia, the average time from the initiation of anticoagulation to becoming symptom-free is 7 months [6].

Literature Review

When evaluating patients with osteonecrosis, particularly multifocal, physicians should first differentiate between osteonecrosis secondary to high-dose long-term corticosteroids, alcoholism, fracture dislocation, etc., and primary ("idiopathic") osteonecrosis. We believe that thrombophilia, hypofibrinolysis [13–16], and eNOS-mediated abnormalities of nitric oxide metabolism [17, 18] play important roles in the pathogenesis of idiopathic osteonecrosis.

We have noted that when compared to normal controls, consecutively referred patients with idiopathic osteonecrosis are more likely to have familial thrombophilia including heterozygosity for the factor V Leiden mutation, high factor VIII, high homocysteine, and high anticardiolipin antibody IgM (Table 1.1).

Patients with osteonecrosis secondary to steroids, alcohol excess, trauma, etc., are marginally more likely ($p = .059$) than normal controls to have factor V Leiden heterozygosity, as well as high homocysteine, anticardiolipin antibody IgM, and low antigenic free protein S (Table 1.1).

The natural history of untreated, idiopathic osteonecrosis of the hip is 20–50 % hip survival within a 2-year follow-up period [19]. Mont et al. [20] concluded "…while small medially located lesions have a low rate of progression, the natural history of asymptomatic, medium-sized, and especially large, osteonecrotic lesions is progression in a substantial number of patients." In subjects with idiopathic osteonecrosis and familial thrombophilia-hypofibrinolysis, provided that anticoagulant therapy is started before segmental collapse of the involved bone (Ficat stages I or II), osteonecrosis may be arrested or even reversed [5, 12, 13]. There were 6200 total hip replacements in the USA for osteonecrosis in 2008 [21]. Diagnosis of medically treatable etiologies of osteonecrosis before bone collapse has been shown to reduce the incidence of total hip and knee replacement [5, 6, 12, 22].

The pathogenesis of osteonecrosis (ON) probably reflects a "multiple etiology" [23] model. We [13], and then others [14], have postulated a sequence for development of ON: venous thrombosis due to thrombophilia-hypofibrinolysis causes osseous venous outflow obstruction, leading to increased intraosseous venous pressure, reduced arterial flow, ischemia, and bone death. Experimental models of ON [24] confirm venous occlusion as the primary event.

Primary (idiopathic) ON of hips and knees [25] in adults [3] and Legg-Calve-Perthes (LCP) in children [26, 27] is commonly associated with thrombophilia-hypofibrinolysis. Factor V Leiden heterozygosity and high anticardiolipin antibody (ACLA) IgG and IgM are associated with LCP in childhood [26]. In adults, relationships have been described between ON and factor V Leiden heterozygosity [28], hypofibrinolysis [18], or reduction of nitric oxide (NO) production by the T-786C mutation of the endothelial nitric oxide synthase gene (eNOS) [18].

The association of heritable thrombophilia-hypofibrinolysis with ON is important because the diagnosis provides a medical (anticoagulation) approach to decrease the frequency of total

Clinical Pearls and Pitfalls

- In the presence of major gene thrombophilia [6, 12, 13], particularly factor V Leiden or prothrombin gene heterozygosity, exogenous estrogen or (particularly) testosterone appears to interact with the heritable thrombophilia, leading to deep venous thrombosis, pulmonary embolus, and osteonecrosis [4, 10].
- In cases with otherwise idiopathic osteonecrosis of the hip or knee, provided that the exogenous estrogen-testosterone is discontinued and anticoagulation is initiated, usually medical treatment can relieve the pain, allowing normal physical activity, possibly with slow healing of the osteonecrotic bone.

- Familial thrombophilia (factor V Leiden heterozygosity) and hypofibrinolysis (4G4G PAI-1 gene homozygosity) can be associated with multifocal idiopathic osteonecrosis but more commonly with unifocal osteonecrosis (Table 1.1).
- Particularly in the presence of factor V Leiden heterozygosity [6, 12, 13], provided that anticoagulation is started before structural collapse of the bone (Ficat stages I–II), idiopathic osteonecrosis can be stabilized, with resolution of pain and resumption of normal function. Long-term (4–16 years) anticoagulation, initiated in Ficat stages I–II of idiopathic hip osteonecrosis patients with familial thrombophilia, can change the natural history of osteonecrosis, stopping progression, resolving pain, and restoring function [6].
- Because there is also a definite association between coagulation disorders and secondary osteonecrosis (Table 1.1), the patient's history is very important, since anticoagulation initiated in Ficat stages I–II of secondary osteonecrosis does not appear to alter the course of the disease [5].
- In those patients with Ficat stages III and IV osteonecrosis, although anticoagulation cannot forestall the need for total joint replacement, presurgical determination of thrombophilia-hypofibrinolysis identifies patients at high risk for postoperative deep venous thrombosis-pulmonary embolism for whom vigorous postoperative thromboprophylaxis would be particularly important [29–32].
- In patients hetero-or homozygous for the T786C eNOS mutation, addition of 9 g/day of over the counter L-Arginine [33] may slow progression of osteonecrosis [34].

hip replacement (THR) and total knee replacement [6, 12, 13]. We speculate that enoxaparin can stop the progression of Ficat stages I and II primary ON of the femoral head by facilitating lysis of intraosseous thrombi, allowing bone healing [5, 6].

References

1. Glueck CJ, Freiberg R, Tracy T, Stroop D, Wang P. Thrombophilia and hypofibrinolysis: pathophysiologies of osteonecrosis. Clin Orthop. 1997;334:43–56.
2. Mannucci PM, Franchini M. Classic thrombophilic gene variants. Thromb Haemost. 2015;114:885–9.
3. Bjorkman A, Svensson PJ, Hillarp A, Burtscher IM, Runow A, Benoni G. Factor V leiden and prothrombin gene mutation: risk factors for osteonecrosis of the femoral head in adults. Clin Orthop Relat Res. 2004;425:168–72.
4. Glueck CJ, Riaz R, Prince M, Freiberg RA, Wang P. Testosterone therapy interacts with previously undiagnosed familial thrombophilia, facilitating development of osteonecrosis. Orthopedics. 2015;38:e1073–8.
5. Glueck CJ, Freiberg RA, Sieve L, Wang P. Enoxaparin prevents progression of stages I and II osteonecrosis of the hip. Clin Orthop Relat Res. 2005;435:164–70.
6. Glueck CJ, Freiberg RA, Wissman R, Wang P. Long term anticoagulation (4–16 years) stops progression of idiopathic hip osteonecrosis associated with familial thrombophilia. Adv Orthop. 2015;2015:138382.
7. Touma L, Filion KB, Atallah R, Eberg M, Eisenberg MJ. A meta-analysis of randomized controlled trials of the risk of bleeding with apixaban versus vitamin K antagonists. Am J Cardiol. 2015;115:533–41.
8. Wasserlauf G, Grandi SM, Filion KB, Eisenberg MJ. Meta-analysis of rivaroxaban and bleeding risk. Am J Cardiol. 2013;112:454–60.
9. Bloom BJ, Filion KB, Atallah R, Eisenberg MJ. Meta-analysis of randomized controlled trials on the risk of bleeding with dabigatran. Am J Cardiol. 2014;113:1066–74.
10. Freedman J, Glueck CJ, Prince M, Riaz R, Wang P. Testosterone, thrombophilia, thrombosis. Transl Res. 2015;165:537–48.
11. Williamson D, Brown K, Luddington R, Baglin C, Baglin T. Factor V Cambridge: a new mutation (Arg306-->Thr) associated with resistance to activated protein C. Blood. 1998;91:1140–4.
12. Glueck CJ, Freiberg RA, Wang P. Medical treatment of osteonecrosis of the knee associated with thrombophilia-hypofibrinolysis. Orthopedics. 2014;37:e911–6.
13. Glueck CJ Freiberg RA, Wang P. Treatment of osteonecrosis of the hip and knee with enoxaparin. Osteonecrosis, *ed* Koo KH, Mont M, Jones L 2014;Chapter 32, pp 241–247, Berlin Springer.

14. Orth P, Anagnostakos K. Coagulation abnormalities in osteonecrosis and bone marrow edema syndrome. Orthopedics. 2013;36:290–300.
15. Glueck CJ, Freiberg RA, Wang P. Heritable thrombophilia-hypofibrinolysis and osteonecrosis of the femoral head. Clin Orthop Relat Res. 2008;466:1034–40.
16. Glueck CJ, Freiberg RA, Fontaine RN, Tracy T, Wang P. Hypofibrinolysis, thrombophilia, osteonecrosis. Clin Orthop. 2001;386:19–33.
17. Koo KH, Lee JS, Lee YJ, Kim KJ, Yoo JJ, Kim HJ. Endothelial nitric oxide synthase gene polymorphisms in patients with nontraumatic femoral head osteonecrosis. J Orthop Res. 2006;24:1722–8.
18. Glueck CJ, Freiberg RA, Boppana S, Wang P. Thrombophilia, hypofibrinolysis, the eNOS T-786C polymorphism, and multifocal osteonecrosis. J Bone Joint Surg Am. 2008;90:2220–9.
19. Hofmann S, Mazieres B. Osteonecrosis: natural course and conservative therapy. Orthopade. 2000;29:403–10.
20. Mont MA, Zywiel MG, Marker DR, McGrath MS, Delanois RE. The natural history of untreated asymptomatic osteonecrosis of the femoral head: a systematic literature review. J Bone Joint Surg Am. 2010;92:2165–70.
21. Johnson AJ, Mont MA, Tsao AK, Jones LC. Treatment of femoral head osteonecrosis in the United States: 16-year analysis of the Nationwide inpatient sample. Clin Orthop Relat Res. 2014;472:617–23.
22. Glueck CJ, Freiberg RA, Wissman R, Wang P. Long term anticoagulation (4–16 years) stops progression of idiopathic hip osteonecrosis associated with familial thrombophilia. Adv Orthop. 2015;29:1–7.
23. Ficat P. Cortisone associated necrosis of bone. In: Hungerford D, editor. Ischemia and necrosis of bone. Baltimore: Williams and Wilkins; 1980. p. 171–6.
24. Boss JH, Misselevich I. Osteonecrosis of the femoral head of laboratory animals: the lessons learned from a comparative study of osteonecrosis in man and experimental animals. Vet Pathol. 2003;40:345–54.
25. Bjorkman A, Burtscher IM, Svensson PJ, Hillarp A, Besjakov J, Benoni G. Factor V Leiden and the prothrombin 20210A gene mutation and osteonecrosis of the knee. Arch Orthop Trauma Surg. 2005;125:51–5.

26. Balasa VV, Gruppo RA, Glueck CJ, et al. Legg-Calve-Perthes disease and thrombophilia. J Bone Joint Surg Am. 2004;86-A:2642–7.
27. Vosmaer A, Pereira RR, Koenderman JS, Rosendaal FR, Cannegieter SC. Coagulation abnormalities in Legg-Calve-Perthes disease. J Bone Joint Surg Am. 2010;92:121–8.
28. Glueck CJ, Freiberg RA, Boriel G, et al. The role of the factor V leiden mutation in osteonecrosis of the hip. Clin Appl Thromb Hemost. 2013;19:499–503.
29. Westrich GH, Sculco TP. Prophylaxis against venous thrombo-embolic disease: costs and controversy. J Bone Joint Surg Am. 2002;84-A:2306–7.
30. Westrich GH, Weksler BB, Glueck CJ, Blumenthal BF, Salvati EA. Correlation of thrombophilia and hypofibrinolysis with pulmonary embolism following total hip arthroplasty: an analysis of genetic factors. J Bone Joint Surg Am. 2002;84-A:2161–7.
31. Westrich GH, Sanchez PM. Prevention and treatment of thromboembolic disease: an overview. Instr Course Lect. 2002;51:471–80.
32. Mont MA, Jones LC, Rajadhyaksha AD, et al. Risk factors for pulmonary emboli after total hip or knee arthroplasty. Clin Orthop Relat Res. 2004;422:154–63.
33. Glueck CJ, Valdes A, Bowe D, Munsif S, Wang P. The endothelial nitric oxide synthase T-786c mutation, a treatable etiology of Prinzmetal's angina. Transl Res. 2013;162:64–6.
34. Glueck CJ, Freiberg RA, Oghene J, Fontaine RN, Wang P. Association between the T-786C eNOS polymorphism and idiopathic osteonecrosis of the head of the femur. J Bone Joint Surg Am. 2007;89:2460–8.

Chapter 2
Bisphosphonates

Hamed Vahedi and Javad Parvizi

Case Presentation

A 38-year-old female presented to the office because of an ongoing left-sided hip pain for the past 4 months. The patient had a mild antalgic limp and walked with the help of a cane. She complained of intermittent pain radiating to the left groin and anterior medial thigh region. She stated that her symptoms were aggravated by walking and stair climbing. Her pain was relieved by sitting and resting. The patient had previously sought medical advice and was prescribed nonsteroidal anti-inflammatory medications.

H. Vahedi, MD
Rothman Institute at Thomas Jefferson University,
Philadelphia, PA, USA

J. Parvizi, MD, FRCS (✉)
James Edwards Professor of Orthopaedic Surgery, Sidney Kimmel
School of Medicine, Rothman Institute at Thomas Jefferson
University, Sheridan Building, Suite 1000, 125 S 9th Street,
Philadelphia, PA 19107, USA
e-mail: parvj@aol.com

R.J. Sierra (ed.), *Osteonecrosis of the Femoral Head*,
DOI 10.1007/978-3-319-50664-7_2,
© Mayo Foundation for Medical Education and Research 2017

19

Diagnosis/Assessment

On physical exam, range of motion of the left hip was 110° of flexion, 30° of internal rotation, and 40° of external rotation and most pain being felt in abduction and internal rotation. FABER test was positive. She had no pertinent medical history or risk factors for osteonecrosis of the femoral head (ONFH). Radiographs and MRI (Figs. 2.1 and 2.2) confirmed the presence of ONFH of the left hip. The joint space appeared to be excellent with no evidence of collapse of the articular cartilage. The patient was thought to have Ficat II ONFH of the left hip.

Management

Surgical and nonsurgical options were discussed with the patient. One of the nonsurgical options offered to her was administration of bisphosphonate medications. She opted to

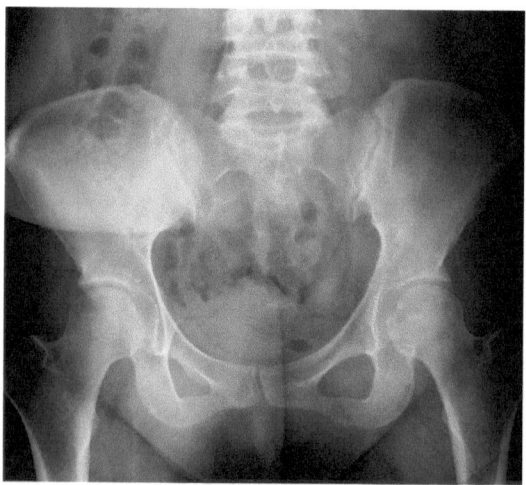

Figure 2.1 Osteonecrosis of the femoral head of *left* hip with good joint space and no evidence of collapse or flattening

receiving the bisphosphonate treatment. She was prescribed 70 mg of alendronate weekly. The bisphosphonates appeared to provide some degree of pain relief, and she was content with the management.

Outcome

The ONFH unfortunately progressed, resulting in collapse of the femoral head and ensuing arthritis (Figs. 2.3 and 2.4). Thus, after 8 months of being on bisphosphonate treatment, patient underwent total hip arthroplasty.

Literature Review

There are several studies reporting on the use of Bps for treatment of ONFH. Young-Kyun Lee et al. reported the results of their prospective, randomized, multicenter study on 110 patients with

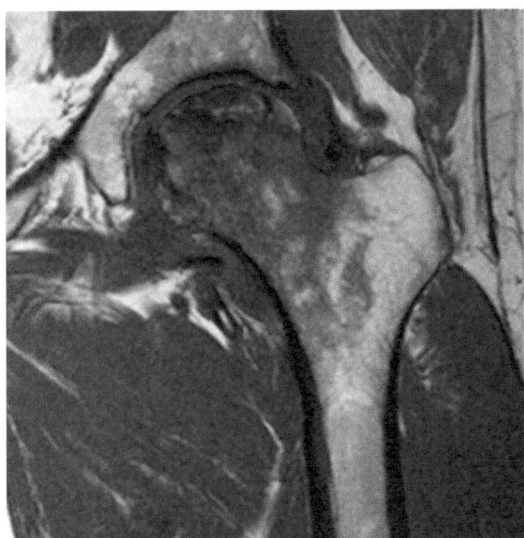

FIGURE 2.2 *Left* hip MRI showing ONFH and bone marrow edema

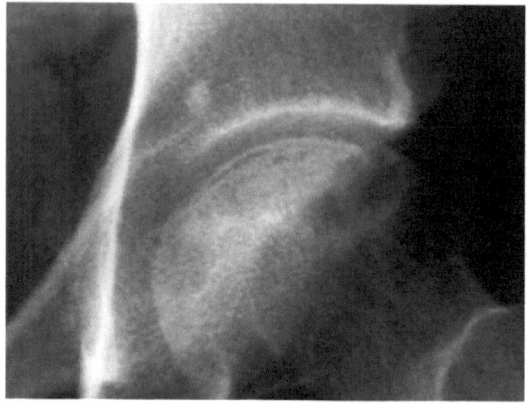

FIGURE 2.3 Femoral head collapse and the crescent sign after 8 months of treatment with bisphosphonates

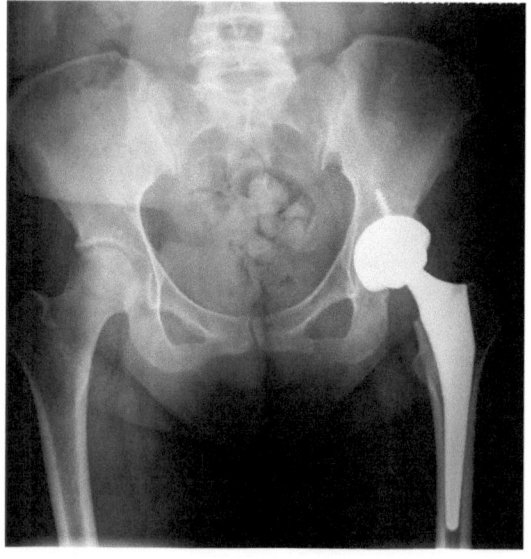

FIGURE 2.4 *Left* total hip arthroplasty after patient developed collapse of the femoral head and ensuing arthritis

Steinberg stage 1 or 2 nontraumatic ONFH with a necrotic area of >30% [1]. Patients in case group received 5 mg of zoledronate, intravenously per year for 2 years, and observed for a minimum of 2 years after enrollment. During 2 years follow-up, 29 femoral heads in zoledronate group and 22 in control group underwent THA. They concluded that zoledronate for Steinberg stage 1 or 2 ONFH with a medium to large necrotic area did not prevent the collapse of the femoral head or reduce the need for THA [1].

Kuo-An Lai et al. reported the results of the use of alendronate in 40 patients (54 hips) with Steinberg stage 2 and 3 with necrotic area >30% in a randomized clinical study. Patients took 70 mg alendronate per week for 25 weeks, and the minimum follow-up was 24 months. Only 2 of 29 femoral heads in the alendronate group collapsed compared to the collapse of 19 out of 25 femoral heads in the control group [2].

Agarwala et al. reported the 10-year follow-up of 40 patients (53 hips) with Ficat stages 1, 2, and 3 ONFH treated with alendronate for 3 years. THA was needed in seven hips, five of whom had stage 3 disease at the time of enrollment. Ten of the 34 hips that were in pre-collapse stage at the onset of study had collapsed during the 10-year follow-up (indicating a failure rate of 29%). They concluded that long-term outcome supported the use of alendronate as a valuable modality for treatment of ONFH, regardless of the stage of the disease [3].

Agarwala et al. presented a clinical and radiological analysis of 395 patients with Ficat stages 1, 2, and 3 ONFH who were treated with oral alendronate for 3 years with a mean follow-up of 4 years [4]. Collapse of the femoral head and arthritis ensued resulting in the need for THA in 4 of 215 (2%) of stage 1 hips, 10 of 129 (8%) hips with stage 2, and 17 of 51 (33%) hips with stage 3 disease. Their results showed an improvement in the clinical function, a reduction in the rate of collapse, and a decrease in the requirement for THA for patients who received Bps treatment. Even in patients with Ficat stage 3 ONFH, some benefit was obtained from treatment with alendronate by at least delaying the need for THA.

Clinical Pearls and Pitfalls

- Bps may be a viable option for treatment and potentially for prevention of progression of the ONFH in symptomatic patients. The literature suggests that the type, dose, duration, and mode of administration of the Bps may influence the outcome. In addition, there may be individual variations in the response with some patients with ONFH responding to the treatment better than others.
- At our institution, we use weekly or monthly oral protocol (70 mg of alendronate per week or 150 mg ibandronate per month). We also believe it is important that patients receiving Bps should also be administered supplemental calcium and vitamin D, especially in those with inadequate dietary intake. It is important to note that calcium supplements should not be taken within 60 min of ibandronate sodium administration, as coadministration may interfere with the absorption of ibandronate sodium.
- We prefer to avoid bisphosphonates in patients with abnormalities of the esophagus which delay esophageal emptying such as stricture and achalasia, inability to stand or sit upright for at least 30 min, hypocalcemia, hypersensitivity to the product, and atrial fibrillation.

References

1. Lee Y-K, Young-Chan HA, et al. Does zoledronate prevent femoral head collapse from osteonecrosis? J Bone Joint. 2015;97(14):1142–8.
2. Lai K-A, Shen W-J, et al. The use of alendronate to prevent early collapse of the femoral head in patients with nontraumatic osteonecrosis. JBone Joint. 2005;87(10):2155–9.

3. Agarwala S, Satyajit B. Shah Ten-year follow-up of avascular necrosis of femoral head treated with alendronate for 3 years. J Arthroplasty. 2011;26(7):1128–34.
4. Agarwala S, Shah S, Joshi VR. The use of alendronate in the treatment of avascular necrosis of the femoral head. J Bone Joint (Br). 2009;91-B:1013–8.

Chapter 3
Successful Decompression with Multiple Percutaneous Drilling

Todd P. Pierce, Julio J. Jauregui, Jeffrey J. Cherian, Randa K. Elmallah, and Michael A. Mont

Case Presentation

An 18-year-old man with a history of T-cell non-Hodgkin's lymphoma presented with a 10-month history of bilateral hip pain. He had undergone a course of high-dose corticosteroids as part of the treatment regimen for his malignancy. He has a past medical history of a left subclavian deep vein thrombosis and a pulmonary embolism.

T.P. Pierce, MD • J.J. Jauregui, MD • J.J. Cherian, DO
R.K. Elmallah, MD • M.A. Mont, MD (✉)
Center for Joint Preservation and Replacement, Rubin Institute for Advanced Orthopaedics, Sinai Hospital of Baltimore, 2401 West Belvedere Avenue, Baltimore, MD 21215, USA
e-mail: tpierce@gwmail.gwu.edu; juljau@gmail.com; jjaicherian@gmail.com; randaelmallah@gmail.com; mmont@lifebridgehealth.org; rhondamont@aol.com

R.J. Sierra (ed.), *Osteonecrosis of the Femoral Head*, 27
DOI 10.1007/978-3-319-50664-7_3,
© Mayo Foundation for Medical Education and Research 2017

Diagnosis/Assessment

Radiographs confirmed right hip Ficat stage II. On examination, he had normal muscle tone and strength (see Fig. 3.1a, b).

Management

After consultation with the patient regarding the risks, benefits, and alternatives of various treatment options, it was decided that he would undergo right hip decompression with multiple drill holes.

Core Decompression

After adequate spinal anesthesia, we prepared and draped the right hip in the usual aseptic manner. We used a 3.4

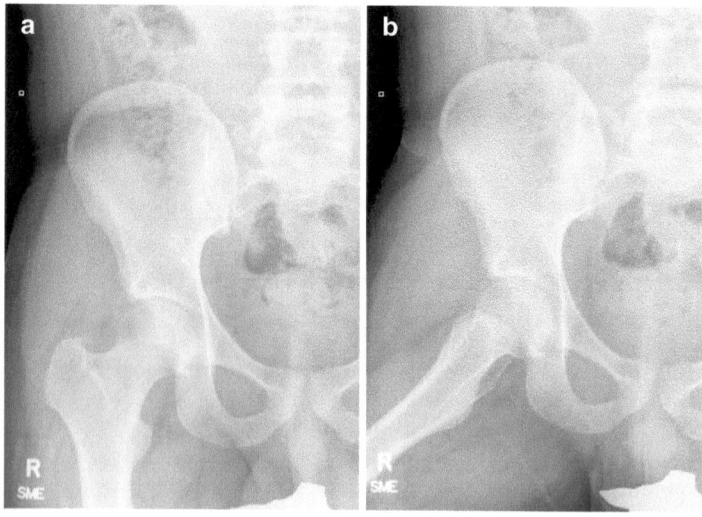

FIGURE 3.1 (**a**, **b**) Preoperative radiographs showing Ficat stage II cystic lesion

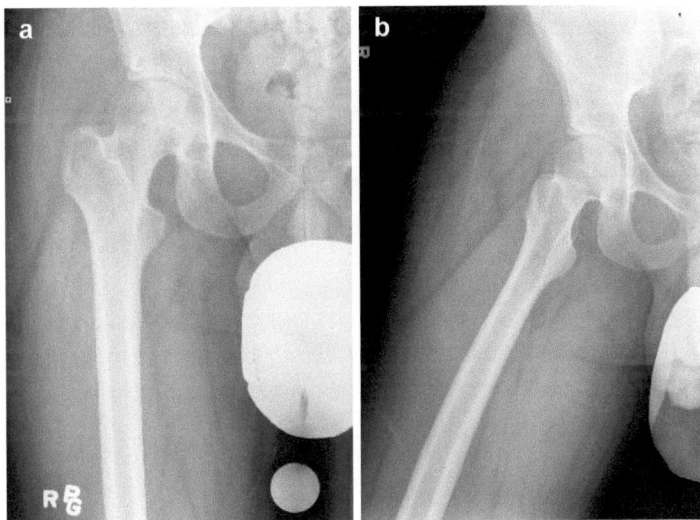

FIGURE 3.2 (**a, b**) Post-decompression and lightbulb grafting radiographs showing no signs of disease progression

drill bit, and under fluoroscopic control, looking at both anteroposterior (AP) and lateral views, using one entrance hole laterally, we made two passes distal to the greater trochanter into the right hip targeting the lesion. The wound was then covered with a sterile dressing, and the patient was brought back to the recovery room in a stable condition. He was discharged with instructions to bear 50% of weight on the right. At 6-week follow-up, he was advanced to full weight bearing.

Outcome

The patient was followed for 10 years (1, 2, 5, and 10 years post-decompression), and radiographs obtained at latest follow-up showed no evidence of any collapse of the femoral head, fracture, or dislocation (see Fig. 3.2). He had no complaints, minimal to no discomfort, and full range of motion in his hip.

TABLE 3.1 Outcomes of multiple drill-hole decompression

Author, year	Number of hips	Mean number of passes (range)	Stage	Mean follow-up, months (range)	Hip survival rate, %
Al Amran A. [1], 2013	33	–	Ficat I and II	38 (37–127)	88
Kang et al. [2], 2012	81	–	Ficat II	63 (48–75)	85
Song et al. [3], 2006	120	12 (4–22)	Ficat I and II	87 (60–134)	78
Mont et al. [4], 2004	45	– (2–3)	Steinberg I	24 (20–39)	80

Literature Review

Core decompression in the literature has been seen as most effective when performed in the earliest pre-collapse stages of ON. Furthermore, more recent studies have shown better outcomes than older studies. This may be due to a surgical technique which involves drilling multiple holes, which has shown positive results (see Table 3.1).

Due to the concern regarding the risk of subtrochanteric fractures with traditional core decompressions, this technique has gained popularity among practitioners. It is recommended that at least two passes be made for small- and medium-sized lesions, while a minimum of three passes should be performed for large-sized ones.

Clinical Pearls and Pitfalls

- The most ideal patient for this procedure would be one with pre-collapse disease with a small- to medium-sized lesion (based on Kerboul angle measurements).
  - Large, greater than 200°
  - Medium, 161–199°
  - Small, less than 160°

- It is important to minimize the risk of subtrochan-
  teric fractures. This can be done by:
  - Ensuring that the drill hole starts above the
    level of the lesser trochanter
  - Using the primary drill hole when adjusting the
    trajectory of the pin
  - Not making a drill hole adjacent to the primary
    hole

- Minimize the risk of skin-edge necrosis when drilling
  with the Steinmann pin by keeping saline-soaked
  gauze at the skin-pin junction during drilling.
- Be cautious when drilling through the osteonecrotic
  lesion as some areas of sclerotic bone may be
  encountered. Forcefully pushing through these areas
  may lead to passing through the femoral head into
  the articular cartilage. If you violate the articular
  cartilage, it is best to convert the patient to a THA.

References

1. Al OA. Multiple drilling compared with standard core decompression for avascular necrosis of the femoral head in sickle cell
   disease patients. Arch Orthop Trauma Surg. 2013;133(5):609.
2. Kang P, Pei F, Shen B, Zhou Z, Yang J. Are the results of multiple
   drilling and alendronate for osteonecrosis of the femoral head
   better than those of multiple drilling? A pilot study. Joint Bone
   Spine. 2012;79(1):67.
3. Song WS, Yoo JJ, Kim YM, Kim HJ. Results of multiple drilling
   compared with those of conventional methods of core decompression. Clin Orthop Relat Res. 2007;454:139.
4. Mont MA, Ragland PS, Etienne G. Core decompression of the
   femoral head for osteonecrosis using percutaneous multiple
   small-diameter drilling. Clin Orthop Relat Res. 2004;429:131.

Chapter 4
Simultaneous Cell Therapy Preserving Surgery and Contralateral Arthroplasty for Bilateral Hip Osteonecrosis

Philippe Hernigou, Arnaud Dubory, Damien Potage, and Charles Henri Flouzat Lachaniette

Case Presentation

A 24-year-old African man presented complaining of vague pains in the left hip in 1992. Physical examination revealed decreased internal rotation with pain on the left side and no pain on right side at hip examination; the patient did not demonstrate any sensory or motor deficits. A pelvis radiograph was normal, and pain was first related to crises.

P. Hernigou, MD (✉) • C.H.F. Lachaniette, MD
Professor of Orthopaedic Surgery, University Paris East,
Department of Orthopaedic Surgery, 51 avenue du Maréchal de
Lattre de Tassigny, 94010 cedex, Créteil, France
e-mail: philippe.hernigou@wanadoo.fr

A. Dubory, MD • D. Potage, MD
University Paris East, Department of Orthopaedic Surgery,
51 avenue du Maréchal de Lattre de Tassigny,
94010 cedex, Créteil, France

R.J. Sierra (ed.), *Osteonecrosis of the Femoral Head*,
DOI 10.1007/978-3-319-50664-7_4,
© Mayo Foundation for Medical Education and Research 2017

33

Diagnosis/Assessment

Six months after his initial presentation, the patient returned to the clinic. At that time, he ambulated with a limp and complained of bilateral hip pain. Examination of the left hip revealed a limited range of motion. Another radiograph was performed with evident osteonecrosis with collapse on left side and normal aspect on the right hip. A subsequent bilateral hip MRI examination allowed measurement of the extent of involvement of the left femoral head while also demonstrating findings consistent with osteonecrosis on the right painful hip. On the right side, there was no collapse and the osteonecrosis was stage I.

Management

The left hip was treated with a total hip arthroplasty. During the same procedure, the right hip was treated with cell therapy, the patient receiving mesenchymal stem cells bone marrow concentrate from the iliac crests in the area of osteonecrosis.

Preparation of the Patient for Surgery

The complication rate for patients with sickle cell disease undergoing orthopedic procedures is significantly higher than that for patients without sickle disease undergoing similar procedures and particularly for total hip arthroplasty. The medical status and attempts to prevent medical complications should be monitored by a specific medical team who has experience in preoperative management of patients with SCD undergoing orthopedic procedures. Part of the routine evaluation of patients with sickle cell disease should include laboratory tests consisting of serial hemoglobin, HbS%, renal function, liver function, and oxygen saturation. Based on these laboratory tests, the need for preoperative transfusion can be determined. Given the frequency of antigen mismatch between mostly Caucasian donors and African-originated recipients, and in an attempt to prevent alloimmunization, we have used, for over 20 years, blood products which are phenotypically typed for ABO, rhesus (Cc, D, Ee), and Kell. We prevent infection before, during, and after surgery. For primary THA, all patients with gallbladder stones had their gallbladder removed before hip surgery because gallbladder infection is a major source of secondary bone infection. Antibiotics (first- and second-generation cephalosporins, 2.5 g per day) were administered during and after surgery (3 days). Furthermore, all the patients had their implants fixed with cement-containing antibiotics (Palacos Genta). Patients had surgery only when white blood cell count, erythrocyte sedimentation rate, and C-reactive protein values were within normal limits (according to the disease). According to the frequency of osteomyelitis in SCD, intraoperatively, aspirates, smears, and excised specimens were collected before antibiotic administration and cultured for growth of aerobic and anaerobic bacilli. Histologic sections were examined for evidence of bacterial infection. After the operation, the antibiotics were continued for 3 days if intraoperative cultures were negative and for 1 month if the cultures or histologic examination were positive.

Surgical Technique

Each patient underwent hip-preserving surgery at the same time that THA surgery was performed. Patients were placed on lateral position when THA surgery was performed, and posterolateral approach was used. Under general anesthetic, surgery was performed in three periods of times (first time, mesenchymal stem cell aspiration from bone marrow; second time, hip arthroplasty; third time, injection of MSCs in the contralateral hip).

Mesenchymal stem cell aspiration from bone marrow was first performed: bone marrow harvesting was done on the posterior iliac crest before hip arthroplasty incision and after installation of the patient for hip arthroplasty. The marrow was aspirated in small fractions as previously described, to reduce the degree of dilution by peripheral blood. Several perforations (between three and five) were made through the same skin opening. Each perforation into the posterior iliac crest was spaced at approximately 2 cm from the other to avoid dilution by aspiration in the previous hole. All aspirates representing average 150 mL were pooled in plastic bags containing an anticoagulant solution (citric acid, sodium citrate, dextrose). The buffy coat containing progenitor cells was concentrated during the time of the arthroplasty.

Hip arthroplasty: We used a posterolateral approach and general anesthesia with meticulous control of oxygenation and hydration. Patient received the same implant as used for osteonecrosis related to other causes or for osteoarthritis. The prostheses were manufactured by Ceraver (Ceraver Osteal, Roissy, France). The stem was made of anodized titanium alloy (TiAl6V4) and was smooth and cemented. The ceramic head was 32 mm in diameter and anchored through a Morse taper. The acetabular component was a cemented polyethylene cup. Difficulty observed during surgery was avoiding femoral perforation in relation to areas of dense bony sclerosis with complete obliteration of the medullary canal and with abnormalities in the femoral version. Technical difficulty on the acetabulum was related to the bone that was usually soft with isolated areas of dense bone that could lead to eccentric reaming. The patient received postoperative thromboembolic prophylaxis for 30 days.

MSCs supercharged in the contralateral osteonecrosis: After hip arthroplasty, the patient was placed on the supine position for the hip cell therapy preserving surgery. Patient was placed on a table with two image intensifiers with a C arm. We sterilized the skin with the operated hip placed at 90° hip and knee flexion and internally adducted the hip. When sterilization was done, a sterilized drape was covered below the sterilized skin. Sterilized drapes were whisked on the sterilized area, and the foot was packed with a sterilized drape and fixed with sterilized bandage to allow internal rotation of the hip during the procedure. The bone marrow injection is done with a percutaneous approach using a 3 mm diameter trephine (trocar of Mazabraud, Collin, France). The instrument is introduced through the greater trochanter, as in conventional core decompression. Its position in the femoral head and in the necrotic segment is monitored with biplane fluoroscopy. Since, at the time of treatment, the plain radiographs will show little if any evidence of necrosis, the preoperative MRI scans should be used together with the image intensifier views, to determine the site of the lesion. To avoid unrecognized joint penetration that may occur because radiograph beam projects an equatorial dimension of the femoral head on to the film, the femur head should be rotated in the acetabulum to obtain various radiographic incidences of the head, or, conversely, the screen intensifier may be rotated around the femur head to examine its contours and prevent "blind" spots. It should, however, be borne in mind that the rotation of the screen intensifier in a single plane reduces the "blind" zones but does not completely eradicate them. The bone marrow is injected slowly (20 cc during 2 min) into the femoral head.

Outcome

Currently, the patient is at 22 years follow-up; the right hip is normal both clinically and on MRI. The left hip treated with total hip arthroplasty had revision in 2010 for PE cup loosening, osteolysis, and wear. The patient received postoperative thromboembolic prophylaxis for 30 days. Full weight bearing was allowed and possible without crutches after 1 week. It is interesting to note that at the most recent follow-up (>20 years), the preserved hip by cell therapy is pain-free with an MRI demonstrating total regression of the osteonecrosis, while the left hip with arthroplasty had revision. THA in SCD involves a higher complication rate incidence of failure with revision than arthroplasty in osteonecrosis related to other conditions. Other surgical options exist for early stages of this disease: core decompression and physical therapy, vascularized grafts (here contraindicated due to the risk of vascular thrombosis related to SCD), and bone marrow transplantation. These treatments should be recommended at early stages of osteonecrosis to postpone the need for THA.

Literature Review

Disease Presentation: Sickle Cell Disease

Literature suggests that sickle cell disease concerns 0.74% of the births in sub-Saharan Africa. By comparison, approximately 0.15% of the black population in the United States and Europe is afflicted with SCD. Sickle cell disease is also an important cause of osteonecrosis affecting persons in the Indian subcontinent, in the Persian Gulf, in South America, and in the Mediterranean countries and those from the Caribbean and Central America. SCD is prevalent in other ethnic groups as well, including those from Mediterranean countries such as North Africa, Turkey, Spain, and Italy. Diagnosis of sickle cell disease is based on analysis of hemoglobin. Typically, this analysis involves protein electrophoresis, although hemoglobin mass spectrometry and DNA analysis are being increasingly used because these techniques enable high-throughput testing. The term sickle cell disease is used to refer to all the different genotypes that cause the characteristic clinical syndrome, whereas sickle cell anemia, the most common form of sickle cell disease, refers specifically to homozygosity for the βS allele. In populations of African ethnic origin, sickle cell anemia typically accounts for 70% of cases of sickle cell disease, with most of the remainder having hemoglobin SC disease (HbSC disease) owing to the coinheritance of the βS and βC alleles. The third major type of sickle cell disease occurs when βS is inherited with a β-thalassemia allele, causing HbS/β-thalassemia. This patient had genotype SC, this genotype giving osteonecrosis at an adult age more frequently than genotype SS giving rather osteonecrosis in children or adolescents. The patients who have SCD have a high risk of bone osteonecrosis due to microvascular occlusion in relation with the disturbance in the erythrocyte architecture, the polymerization of hemoglobin S (in a deoxygenated state) producing cells that are crescent- or sickle-shaped with decreased deformability; the decreased deformability results in greater risk for clotting in small vessels.

Clinical Presentation of the Patient

The prevalence of osteonecrosis in patients with sickle cell disease is as high as 37–50%. Osteonecrosis most commonly occurs in the humeral and femoral heads, due to their limited arterial network, which can easily succumb to occlusion by sickled cells. In both the hip and shoulder joints, the disease is bilateral in approximately 30% of patients. Collapse of the femoral head tends to occur early and at a high rate within 5 years after the diagnosis. No significant risk factors that could cause collapse, such as stage or size, are identified possibly because the rate of collapse is so high. This suggests that conservative operative procedures should be instituted early to try to prevent a poor outcome in hips with stage I or stage II disease. The unfavorable outcome for most patients with an asymptomatic hip and symptomatic osteonecrosis of the femoral head in the contralateral hip related to sickle cell disease suggests that careful screening of the asymptomatic hip should be performed on a regular basis. We recommend that the asymptomatic hip be screened at 6-month intervals after presentation of the symptomatic hip, particularly when there has been collapse of the contralateral hip, because these two factors have been found to be associated with the rate of clinical and radiographic progression in the asymptomatic hip. We also recommend evaluating the patient as soon as possible after the onset of pain because symptoms always preceded collapse. The intervals between the onset of pain and collapse may be as short as 3 months, and for this patient's left hip, time between pain and collapse was 6 months.

Rationale for cell-based strategies in avascular osteonecrosis is to enhance tissue repair; autologous mesenchymal stem cells represent a highly promising candidate among several options for cell-based therapeutic approaches. Adult mesenchymal stromal cells can be isolated from bone marrow. These cells have the multipotential capacity for differentiation into osteoblasts. Bone marrow-derived mononuclear cells also promote formation of new blood vessels due to the presence of endothelial cell progenitors or hemangioblasts in the bone marrow concentrate. Angiogenesis may be promoted both by the increased supply of progenitor cells and angiogenic cytokines produced by the bone marrow cells. MSCs also can release a variety of growth factors to facilitate tissue regeneration in the microenvironment. Thus, the multiple capabilities of MSCs, including their homing ability to injury sites and their paracrine secretions enhancing cell migration, differentiation, and angiogenesis, make them an ideal cell type to mimic a bone autograft by demonstrating all of the key components required for bone repair in osteonecrosis. The bone marrow also contains endothelial progenitors. Their role in angiogenesis and neovascularization has been studied extensively, and positive effects on blood vessel formation after transplantation have been reported.

Clinical Pearls and Pitfalls

- Many patients with bilateral ONFH could suffer from various stages. For the end-stage hip, THA is indicated to be performed for obtaining pain relief and hip function recovery.
- If the contralateral hip seems to be not as serious as the replaced hip, the contralateral hip is indicated to perform hip-preserving surgery to protect the femoral head from collapsing.
- When performing hip-preserving surgery with large-diameter core decompression or with vascularized fibular grafting in one hip and concurrent one-stage total hip arthroplasty (THA) in the contralateral side for bilateral ONFH patients, the patient is asked to remain without weight bearing on the hip-preserving

side and cannot enjoy the immediate benefit of hip arthroplasty. With this technique "simultaneous cell therapy preserving surgery and contralateral arthroplasty for bilateral hip osteonecrosis" that we had performed in more than 300 patients with osteonecrosis during the last 20 years, we allow full weight bearing on both sides after 1 week. Due to the small size of the trocar, the young age of the patient, and the pain relief on both sides, the patient is usually able to walk without crutches after 1 week. Onestage bilateral hip surgery reveals several advantages for these patients with sickle cell disease (but also for patients with other causes of osteonecrosis) compared to two-stage surgery, such as fewer complications related to surgery and anesthesia, lower cost for patients, and shorter inhospital length of stay.

Bibliography

1. Chung SM, Ralston EL. Necrosis of the femoral head associated with sickle-cell anemia and its genetic variants. A review of the literature and study of thirteen cases. J Bone Joint Surg Am. 1969;51:33–58.
2. Diggs LW. Bone and joint lesions in sickle-cell disease. Clin Orthop Relat Res. 1967;52:119–43.
3. Garden MS, Grant RE, Jebraili S. Perioperative complications in patients with sickle cell disease. An orthopedic perspective. Am J Orthop. 1996;25:353–6.
4. Hernigou P, Galacteros F, Bachir D, Goutallier D. Deformities of the hip in adults who have sickle-cell disease and had avascular necrosis in childhood. A natural history of fifty-two patients. J Bone Joint Surg Am. 1991;73:81–92.
5. Hernigou P, Bachir D, Galacteros F. Avascular necrosis of the femoral head in sickle-cell disease. Treatment of collapse by the injection of acrylic cement. J Bone Joint Surg Br. 1993;75:875–80.
6. Hernigou P, Bernaudin F, Reinert P, Kuentz M, Vernant JP. Bone marrow transplantation in sickle cell disease; effect on osteonecrosis. J Bone Joint Surg. 1997;79-A:1726–30.

7. Hernigou P, Lambotte JC. Bilateral hip osteonecrosis: influence of hip size on outcome. Ann Rheum Dis. 2000;59:817–21.

8. Hernigou P, Beaujean F. Treatment of osteonecrosis with autologous bone marrow grafting. Clin Orthop Relat Res. 2002;405:14–23.

9. Hernigou P, Manicom O, Poignard A, Nogier A, Filippini P, De Abreu L. *core* decompression with marrow stem cells. Oper Tech Orthop. 2004;14(2):68–74.

10. Hernigou P, Habibi A, Bachir D, Galacteros F. The natural history of asymptomatic osteonecrosis of the femoral head in adults with sickle cell disease. J Bone Joint Surg Am. 2006;88(12):2565–72.

11. Hernigou P, Zilber S, Filippini P, Rouard H, Mathieu G, Poignard A. Bone marrow injection in hip osteonecrosis. Tech Orthop. 2008;23:18–25.

12. Hernigou P, Zilber S, Filippini P, Mathieu G, Poignard A, Galacteros F. THA in adult osteonecrosis related to sickle cell disease. Clin Orthop Relat Res. 2008;466(2):300–8.

13. Hernigou P, Flouzat-Lachaniette CH, Delambre J, Poignard A, Allain J, Chevallier N, Rouard H. Osteonecrosis repair with bone marrow cell therapies: state of the clinical art. Bone. 2015;70:102–9.

14. Lih LY, Wong YC, Shih HN. One-stage hip arthroplasty and bone grafting for bilateral femoral head osteonecrosis. Clin Orthop Relat Res. 2009;467(6):1522–8.

15. Marcus ND, Enneking WF, Massam RA. The silent hip in idiopathic aseptic necrosis: treatment by bone-grafting. J Bone Joint Surg Am. 1973;55(7):1351–66.

16. Mont MA, Hungerford DS. Non-traumatic avascular necrosis of the femoral head. J Bone Joint Surg Am. 1995;77:459–74.

17. Steinberg MH, Nagel RL, Higgs D. Disorders of hemoglobin: genetics, pathophysiology, and clinical management. New York, NY; Cambridge University Press; 2001. Steinberg MH. Management of sickle cell disease. N Engl J Med. 1999;340:1021–30.

18. Urbaniak JR, Coogan PG, Gunneson EB, Nunley JA. Treatment of osteonecrosis of the femoral head with free vascularized fibular grafting. A long-term follow-up study of one hundred and three hips. J Bone Joint Surg Am. 1995;77(5):681–94.

19. Vichinsky EP, Neumayr LD, Haberkem C, et al. The perioperative complication rate of orthopedic surgery in sickle cell disease: report of the National Sickle Cell Surgery Study Group. Am J Hematol. 1999;62:129–38.

Chapter 5
Bilateral Osteonecrosis Associated with Corticosteroid Treatment: Stem Cell Therapy Versus Core Decompression in the Same Patient

Philippe Hernigou, Arnaud Dubory, Damien Potage, and Charles Henri Flouzat Lachaniette

Case Presentation

A 35-year-old Caucasian man presented complaining of pains in both hips in 1994. The patient had an antalgic limp. He complained of intermittent pain radiating into his right groin and anterior medial thigh region. He

P. Hernigou, MD (✉) • C.H.F. Lachaniette, MD
Professor of Orthopaedic Surgery, University Paris East,
Department of Orthopaedic Surgery, 51 avenue du Maréchal de Lattre de Tassigny, 94010 cedex, Créteil, France
e-mail: philippe.hernigou@wanadoo.fr

A. Dubory, MD • D. Potage, MD
University Paris East, Department of Orthopaedic Surgery,
51 avenue du Maréchal de Lattre de Tassigny,
94010 cedex, Créteil, France

R.J. Sierra (ed.), *Osteonecrosis of the Femoral Head*,
DOI 10.1007/978-3-319-50664-7_5,
© Mayo Foundation for Medical Education and Research 2017

43

stated that his symptoms were aggravated by walking and stair climbing. His pain was relieved by sitting and resting. The patient did not report numbness or paresthesias in his lower extremities. There was no bowel and bladder dysfunction. The patient did not complain of any night sweats, fever, or chills.

The patient had previously sought medical advice and was prescribed painkillers and anti-inflammatories. At that time, he had radiographs of his lumbar spine done which he stated were normal. Subsequently, he had a lumbar spine MRI done. The MRI showed a small disk bulge in the T12/L1 region, but there was no correlation between the patient symptoms and the MRI findings (Fig. 5.1).

Past history revealed that the patient was treated 6 months before with oral corticosteroid therapy during 5 days. The treatment used was a 21-tablet packet of 4-mg methylprednisolone administered in a tapered fashion over a 6-day period. The generic version of the medication was queried, which includes both the generic and proprietary medication (4-mg Medrol Dosepak; Pfizer, New York, New York). The steroid dose in equivalent milligrams of prednisone was 250 mg. The duration of drug therapy was 6 days. The time from administration of steroids to the development of hip symptoms was 6 months.

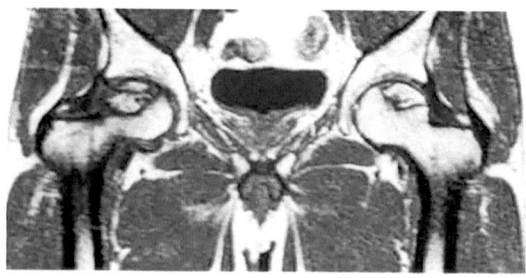

FIGURE 5.1 Preoperative MRI

Diagnosis/Assessment

On physical examination, range of motion of the right hip was severely limited and painful in all ranges, with most pain being felt in abduction and internal rotation. Palpation of the right hip region revealed extreme tenderness. Muscle palpation revealed tenderness in the right thigh and pelvic musculature. Muscle atrophy was also noted in the right thigh musculature. Lumbar spine range of motion was full with end-range pain in right lateral flexion and right rotation. Valsalva was unremarkable. Straight leg raise produced right hip pain. Posterior joint provocation tests were painful for L4 and L5. SI testing was painful for the right sacroiliac joint. Muscle palpation revealed tenderness in the lumbar paraspinal and right gluteal musculature. Muscle palpation revealed tenderness in the right TFL and quadriceps musculature. Lower limb neurological testing revealed normal reflexes and sensory testing bilaterally. Global muscle weakness was noted in the right lower limb when compared to the left.

Despite the low dose of corticosteroids and the delay between the administration and the symptoms in the hip, the patient was suspected as having avascular necrosis of the right hip. He was referred to a medical radiology facility for radiographs of the lumbar spine, right hip, and pelvis. The radiology report stated that the hips were normal (Fig. 5.2).

MR imaging studies were performed with a 1.5-T imager. A set of coronal T1-weighted scout images was then obtained. This first set of coronal T1-weighted images was defined as the limited examination. Pulse sequence parameters were as follows: 450–600/10–15 (repetition time msec/echo time msec), 6-mm section thickness, 2-mm intersection gap, 38-cm field of view, 256×192 matrix, and two signals acquired, which resulted in obtaining 12 images in approximately 3 min 30 s. The presence of osteonecrosis was confirmed on MRI by the presence of a band of low signal intensity in the anterior and superior portion of the femoral head. The percentage of weight-bearing surface involved with avascular necrosis was calculated by dividing the volume of femoral head involved with osteonecrosis by the total volume of the femoral head (Fig. 5.3).

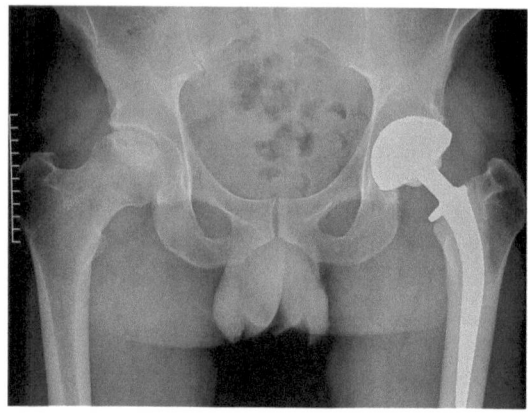

FIGURE 5.2 Radiographs at 5-year follow-up when the patient received arthroplasty on the left hip

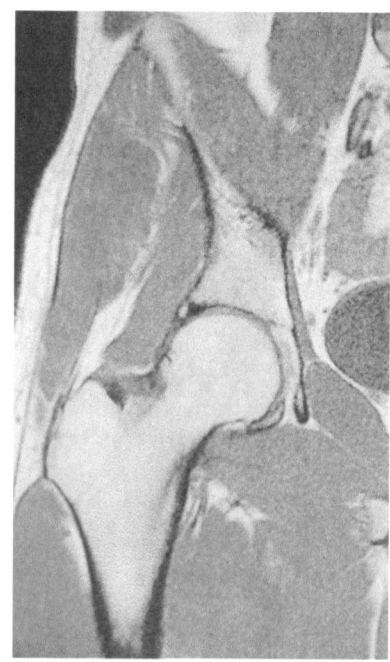

FIGURE 5.3 MRI of the right hip with total repair at the most recent follow-up (20 years)

Management

Both hips were stage I osteonecrosis; the left hip osteonecrosis had the smaller size (15%) compared to the right osteonecrosis (38%). Both hips were treated during the same operative procedure. The left hip with the smaller lesion was treated with core decompression alone, while the right hip was treated with percutaneous injection of bone marrow concentrate.

Operative Technique

Under general anesthesia, the patient was positioned, and both limbs were draped in a sterile sleeve to allow an anteroposterior view and a frog-leg lateral view of both hips. Fluoroscopy was used to visualize the hips. The frog-leg lateral view was obtained with abduction and external rotation of the hip associated with knee flexing.

Core Decompression Alone

A trocar was introduced through the trochanter, as in conventional core decompression with a percutaneous approach using a 4.5-mm diameter trocar (the same trocar used for bone marrow injection – Mazabraud, Collin, France). Its position in the femoral head and in the necrotic zone was monitored with fluoroscopy. The direction of the trocar was adjusted in both planes with anteroposterior and lateral fluoroscopy views. The position of the trocar tip was placed in the osteonecrotic lesion with a separation of 5 mm from adjacent articular cartilage.

Bone Marrow Graft

One hundred and fifty milliliter of marrow was aspirated from the iliac crest. The number of colony-forming unit-fibroblast (CFU-F) was determined from a small aliquot of the bone marrow aspirate after in vitro culturing. CFU-F is used as an indicator of the number of mesenchymal stem cells (MSCs) present, as previously reported (ref). The bone marrow was concentrated as previously reported. Concentrated bone marrow (BMC) was returned to the operating room for injection (20 mL corresponding to 200,000 MSCs) into the femoral head using a trocar with the same diameter as for core decompression alone. During injection, the hip was in internal rotation with the trochanter directed upward. Patients were allowed weight bearing using crutches for the first 10 days and allowed to return to normal activities without crutches after 10 days.

Outcome

At 20-year follow-up, the right hip was pain-free without collapse and total repair on MRI; the left hip after a period of pain relief became again painful at 5-year follow-up, had collapsed, and was operated with THA at 6-year follow-up after core decompression. For the left hip with core decompression alone, the mean volume of repair as determined by MRI at the most recent follow-up was 2 cm³ corresponding to a decrease in the mean ONFH volume from 15 to 13%. For the right hip treated with BMMSCs, the volume of repair evaluated by MRI at the most recent follow-up was 16 cm³ corresponding to a decrease of the mean ONFH volume from 38 to 0%, i.e., a total repair.

Literature Review

Cushing described adverse effects of long-term endogenous hypercortisolism on bone in his 1932 presentation to the Johns Hopkins Medical Society. Eighteen years later, only 1 year after the introduction of cortisone for the treatment of rheumatoid arthritis, clinicians became aware of the rapidly injurious skeletal effects of glucocorticoid administration. Osteoporosis and fractures were clearly recognized as skeletal complications of treatment with cortisone, prednisolone, and prednisone. Collapse of the femoral heads after high-dose therapy was described shortly thereafter. Today, we know that glucocorticoid administration is the most common cause of secondary osteoporosis and one of the leading causes of nontraumatic osteonecrosis. In patients receiving long-term therapy, glucocorticoids induce fractures in 30–50% and osteonecrosis in 9–40%.

This case presentation demonstrates that even a single prescription of short-term, low-dose oral corticosteroid administration is associated with a low but significantly increased risk of being diagnosed with osteonecrosis. Multiple cases of the development of osteonecrosis after short-term, low-dose oral steroid administration have been described. The incidence of glucocorticoid-induced osteonecrosis increases with higher doses and prolonged treatment, although it may occur with short-term exposure. In the Westlaw database, oral doses as low as 290 mg of prednisone and courses that lasted as short as 6 days were held responsible for osteonecrosis (Nash).

Corticosteroids are commonly prescribed to treat many dermatological, respiratory, gastrointestinal, neurologic, and musculoskeletal inflammatory conditions. As a result, corticosteroid use is the most commonly described nontraumatic risk factor for the development of osteonecrosis. The widespread use of oral corticosteroids for these common conditions in often otherwise healthy patients and the potentially devastating sequelae of osteonecrosis after their use can be a source of significant contention and litigation between the patient and prescribing physician. Physicians who prescribe glucocorticoids should educate their patients about side effects and complications including osteoporosis and osteonecrosis, cataract and glaucoma, hypokalemia, hyperglycemia, hypertension, hyperlipidemia, weight gain, fluid retention, easy bruisability, susceptibility to infection, impaired healing, myopathy, adrenal insufficiency, and the steroid withdrawal syndrome. The bone complications are ignored by the majority of specialists who prescribe glucocorticoids, possibly because of the physicians' greater concern for other coexisting disorders, their unfamiliarity with metabolic disorders of the skeleton, or lack of appreciation of the rapidity of the substantial increase in risk of fracture or osteonecrosis. Laboratory testing should include measurement of serum 25-hydroxyvitamin D (25OHD), creatinine, and calcium (in addition to glucose, potassium, and lipids). It is particularly important to check the 25OHD level before the administration of antiresorptive agents to avoid drug-induced hypocalcemia.

Osteonecrosis of the femoral head is a condition with a poor natural history that can be crippling, especially in young active patients. Our series do not provide conclusive proof that there is a cause-effect relation between short-course steroid therapy and osteonecrosis. However, the number of patients seen with this condition in our unit is strong presumptive evidence that some association exists.

Clinical Pearls and Pitfalls

- Patients should be informed of the potential risk of osteonecrosis following the use of steroid medication. Complaints of hip pain in people who have previously been prescribed steroids should produce a high index of suspicion for underlying osteonecrosis of the femoral head. Although early treatment before collapse of the femoral head occurs is beneficial, prevention of this complication is preferable.
- We observed a better outcome in osteonecrotic hip treated with MSCs than in the hip treated with core decompression alone.
- Core decompression (CD) is a widely accepted procedure for treatment of hip osteonecrosis in its early stages (before mechanical failure has occurred). Core decompression can delay the progression of osteonecrosis, but its role in complete reconstruction of the necrotic area is inconsistent. The outcome of CD is not always satisfactory because the reconstruction of the necrotic area by this method may remain

incomplete because of inadequate creeping substitution and bone remodeling. This is attributed to the relative insufficiency of osteoprogenitor cells in the proximal femur of the osteonecrotic hip. The addition of MSCs into the area enriches the cellular environment and augments the biologic repair leading to better healing. Mesenchymal stem cells infiltrated into the necrotic area can potentially augment the biologic repair by differentiating into multiple cell lineages including the osteoprogenitor cells and resulting in bone formation. They also enhance vascularization and oxygen flow to the ischemic tissues and accelerate fracture healing.

Bibliography

1. Cushing H. The basophil adenomas of the pituitary body and their clinical manifestations (pituitary basophilism). Bull Johns Hopkins Hosp. 1932;50:137–95.
2. Boland EW, Headley NE. Management of rheumatoid arthritis with smaller (maintenance) doses of cortisone acetate. JAMA. 1950;144:365–72.
3. Bollet AJ, Black R, Bumin JJ. Major undesirable side-effects resulting from prednisolone and prednisone. JAMA. 1955;157:459–63.
4. Freyberg RH, Traeger CH, Patterson M, et al. Problems of prolonged cortisone treatment for rheumatoid arthritis. JAMA. 1951;147:1538–43.
5. Heiman WG, Freiberger RH. Avascular necrosis of the femoral and humeral heads after high-dosage corticosteroid therapy. N Engl J Med. 1960;263:672–5.
6. Hernigou P, Beaujean F, Lambotte JC. Decrease in the mesenchymal stem-cell pool in the proximal femur in corticosteroid-induced osteonecrosis. J Bone Joint Surg Br. 1999;81(2):349.
7. Hernigou P, Poignard A, Manicom O, et al. The use of percutaneous autologous bone marrow transplantation in nonunion and avascular necrosis of bone. J Bone Joint Surg Br. 2005;87(7):896.

8. Houdek MT, Wyles CC, Packard BD, Terzic A, Behfar A, Sierra RJ. Decreased osteogenic activity of mesenchymal stem cells in patients with corticosteroid-induced osteonecrosis of the femoral head. J Arthroplasty. 2016;31(4):893–8.

9. Lee HS, Huang GT, Chiang H, et al. Multipotent mesenchymal stem cells from femoral bone marrow near the site of osteonecrosis. Stem Cells. 2003;21:190.

10. Liberman JR. Core decompression for osteonecrosis of hip. Clin Orthop. 2004;418:29.

11. LoCascio V, Bonucci E, Imbimbo B, et al. Bone loss in response to long-term glucocorticoid therapy. Bone Miner. 1990;8:39–51.

12. Lorio R, Healy WL, Abramowitz AJ, et al. Clinical outcome and survivorship analysis of core decompression for early osteonecrosis of the femoral head. J Arthroplasty. 1998;13(1):34.

13. Mont MA, Cherian JJ, Sierra RJ, Jones LC, Lieberman JR. Nontraumatic osteonecrosis of the femoral head: where do we stand today? A ten-year update. J Bone Joint Surg Am. 2015;97(19):1604–27.

14. Nash JJ, Nash AG, Leach ME, et al. Medical malpractice and corticosteroid use. Otolaryngol Head Neck Surg. 2011;144:10–5.

15. Pietrogrande V, Mastromarino R. Osteopathia da prolungato trattmento cortisonico. Ortop Tramat. 1957;25:791–810.

16. Weinstein RS. Clinical practice: glucocorticoid-induced bone disease. N Engl J Med. 2011;365:62–70.

17. Wyles CC, Houdek MT, Behfar A, Sierra RJ. Mesenchymal stem cell therapy for osteoarthritis: current perspectives. Stem Cells Cloning. 2015;8:117–24.

Chapter 6
Minimally Invasive Core Decompression Augmented with Concentrated Autologous Mesenchymal Stem Cells

Matthew T. Houdek

Case Presentation

A 19-year-old female presented to our institution complaining of increasing right hip pain for 1 year. She had an underlying diagnosis of vasculitis and idiopathic thrombocytopenic purpura (ITP); because of this she was treated with high-dose oral corticosteroids. Three years prior to her presentation, she underwent an MRI of her abdomen for other reasons which showed changes consistent with ON of her bilateral femoral heads. At that time, she was asymptomatic and chose observation, protected weight bearing, and bisphosphonate therapy. She was unable to tolerate

M.T. Houdek, MD
Department of Orthopaedic Surgery, Mayo Clinic,
Rochester, MN 55905, USA
e-mail: houdek.matthew@mayo.edu

R.J. Sierra (ed.), *Osteonecrosis of the Femoral Head*,
DOI 10.1007/978-3-319-50664-7_6,
© Mayo Foundation for Medical Education and Research 2017

bisphosphonates and weight-bearing restrictions, and over the year prior to her clinic visit, she began to have increasing pain in her right hip. At the time of presentation to our clinic, she was still on daily oral corticosteroids.

Diagnosis/Assessment

On physical exam, she had pain at the end points of internal and external rotation as well as hip flexion. Prior to the procedure, her Harris Hip Score [1] was 69. On AP and frog-leg radiographs, there were no signs of femoral head collapse (Fig. 6.1). In order to assess for progression of the ON, an MRI of both hips was obtained (Fig. 6.2). The MRI showed changes in the subchondral bone consistent with ON. Compared to her preoperative MRI 3 years prior, there

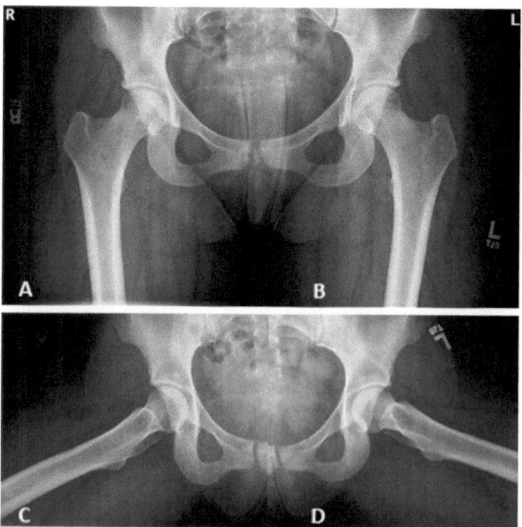

FIGURE 6.1 AP and frog-leg lateral radiographs of the *right* (**a, c**) and *left* (**b, d**) hips showing faint sclerosis of the femoral heads consistent with osteonecrosis; however there were no signs of collapse

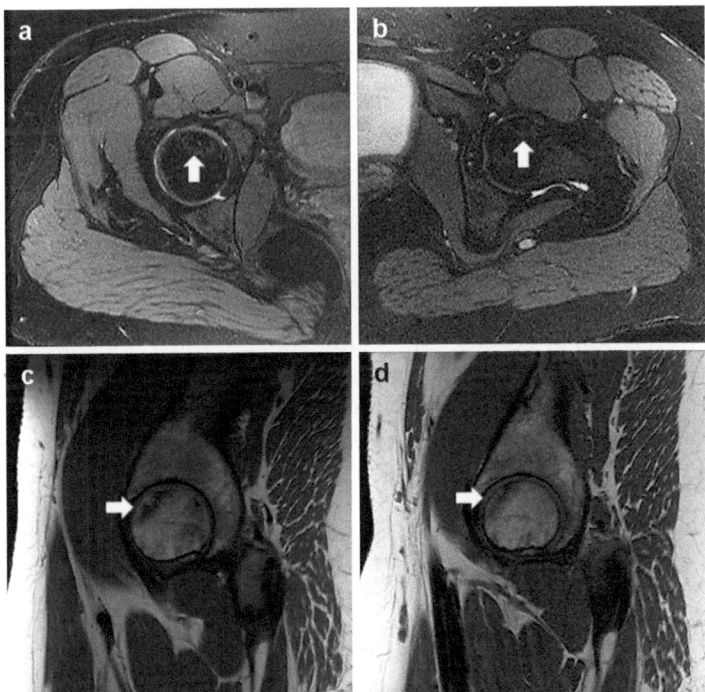

FIGURE 6.2 Axial (**a, b**) and sagittal (**c, d**) MRI images of the right and left hips showing increased signal on T1 (*arrows*, **a, b**) images and decreased intensity on T2 (*arrows*, **c, d**), consistent with features of osteonecrosis. There were no signs of articular cartilage or subchondral collapse

was progression in the size of the ON lesions, especially in the right hip. On the right hip, the necrotic lesion measured 28 mm in maximal dimension and on the left 23 mm in maximal dimension. There was no subchondral collapse.

Management

Due to the increasing pain and her failure of nonoperative treatment modalities, she was offered a bilateral minimally invasive core decompression along with bilateral iliac crest bone marrow concentrate injection. After consultation with the patient regarding the risks, benefits, and alternatives of various treatment options, it was decided that she would undergo this procedure and informed consent was obtained.

Surgical Procedure

The procedure is performed under general anesthesia on a radiolucent table with the patient supine. For the surgical procedure, we use the PerFuse and BioCUE Systems (Fig. 6.3) from Biomet (Biomet Biologics, Warsaw, Indiana). Biplanar fluoroscopy is then used to confirm we are able to obtain appropriate anterior-posterior (AP) and frog-leg lateral images preoperatively. The operative hips and both iliac crests are prepped and draped in the standard fashion.

Bone Marrow Concentration

The procedure is started by obtaining 120 cc of anticoagulated blood. This is typically drawn by anesthesia during the prepping and draping of the patient. The blood is placed into two 60 cc vials and centrifuged for 15 min in the BioCUE System (Biomet Biologics, Warsaw, Indiana). This concentration creates 12 cc of platelet-rich plasma (PRP). The bone marrow is then aspirated from both iliac crests. Over the anterior aspect of the iliac crest, a 2–3-mm incision is made, exposing the iliac crest. The PerFuse trochar (Biomet Biologics) is inserted into each iliac crest between the two tables of the ilium, and the bone marrow is aspirated into 10-mL syringes (Fig. 6.4). This marrow is then concentrated using the BioCUE System (Biomet Biologics). A vial for this system contains 57 cc of bone marrow and 3 cc of heparin. This is concentrated 10×, yielding 6 cc of bone marrow concentrate (BMC). From each crest, we typically obtain 120 cc of bone marrow, yielding 12 cc of BMC. The goal is to obtain 12 cc of BMC for injection into each hip.

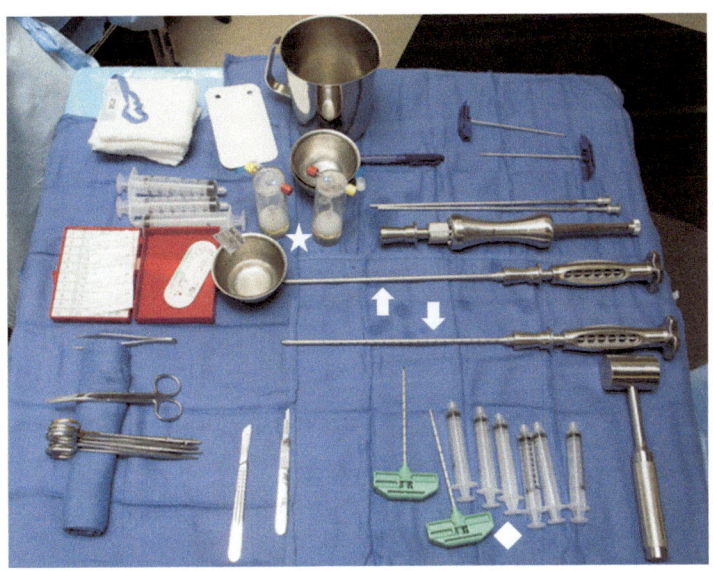

FIGURE 6.3 Surgical table setup showing the PerFuse trochar (*arrows*, Biomet Biologics) and the BioCUE aspirators (*diamond*) and marrow concentrations (*star*, Biomet Biologics) along with a basic orthopedics instrument tray. Additional instruments are not typically necessary

Hip Decompression

During the 15 min that it takes the bone marrow and blood to be centrifuged, we perform the hip decompression. After confirming with fluoroscopy our starting point at the level of the lesser trochanter and distal to the vastus ridge, we make a 1-cm incision over the lateral aspect of the femur just above the tip of the lesser trochanter. The lateral cortex of the femur is then breached by tapping the tip of the decompression trochar into the bone or alternatively with a 3.2-mm drill; the decompression is performed by hand. The 6-mm trochar is advanced from lateral to medial, taking care to check on biplanar fluoroscopy the position of the trochar (Fig. 6.5). The trochar is advanced with gentle mallet taps until the tip is "in" the necrotic lesion which is typically accompanied by a change

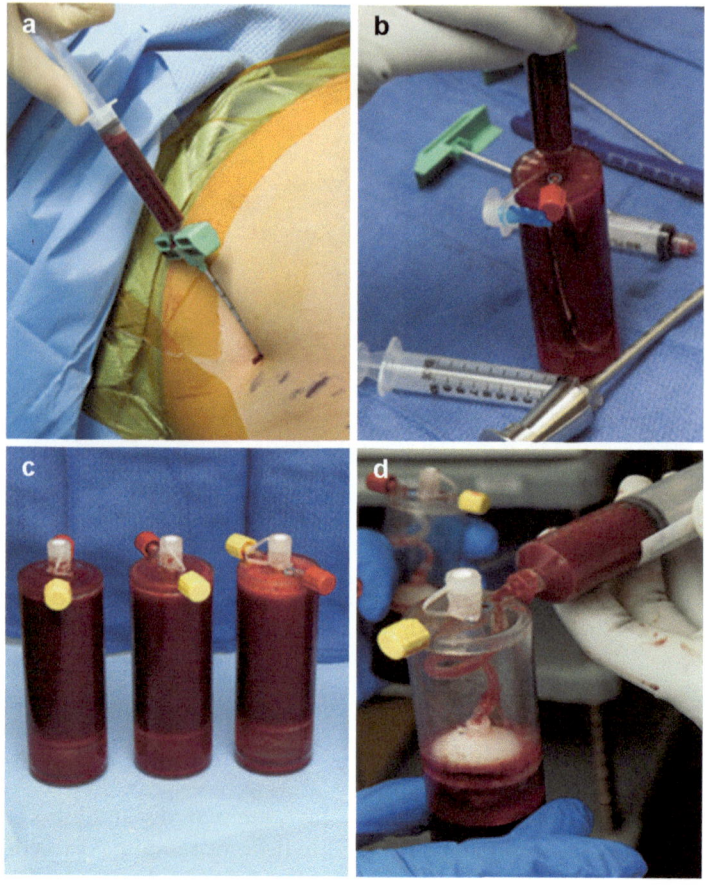

Figure 6.4 The BioCUE aspirators (Biomet Biologics) are used to aspirate bone marrow from the iliac crests (**a**). In cases of bilateral disease, both crests are used. The bone marrow is then injected into the BioCUE concentrators (**b**), for a total of 57 cc of bone marrow and 3 cc of heparin (**c**) to prevent clotting. Once the concentration process is complete, the concentrated bone marrow is then reaspirated (**d**) from the vial for use

in pitch of the mallet strikes. The position is confirmed with biplanar fluoroscopy. It is important that the trochar is not advanced within 5 mm of subchondral bone to avoid collapse. If one cannot visualize the lesion radiographically, the

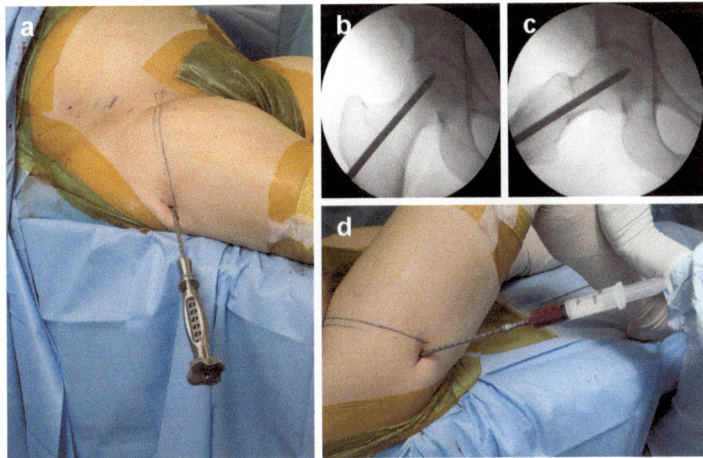

FIGURE 6.5 While the bone marrow is concentrating, a 1-cm incision is made over the lateral thigh. The PerFuse trochar (Biomet Biologics) is then inserted (**a**) at a level below the vastus ridge and above the distal extension of the lesser trochanter. A drill is used to breach the outer cortex; however, the trochar is impacted by hand into the area of osteonecrosis and confirmed on AP (**b**) and frog-leg lateral (**c**) views intraoperatively. Typically, when the area of necrosis is entered, a change in the pitch is heard with the mallet strikes. Once the location is confirmed, the trochar sleeve is removed, the hip is flexed, and the concentrated bone marrow is injected (**d**)

preoperative MRI should be used as a guide as to where the trochar should sit for the decompression.

Injection of Concentrated Bone Marrow

Once the trochar has been confirmed to be in the proper position, the inner sleeve of the trochar is removed, leaving a 6-mm trochar in the area of ON. The hip is then flexed, and the 12 cc of BMC and PRP are then mixed in a 30-cc syringe and injected into the trochar (Fig. 6.5). If there is excessive resistance, the trochar should be retracted to increase the space for the injection while confirming that the tip is in the area of ON. To prevent retrograde, backflow the trochar is removed

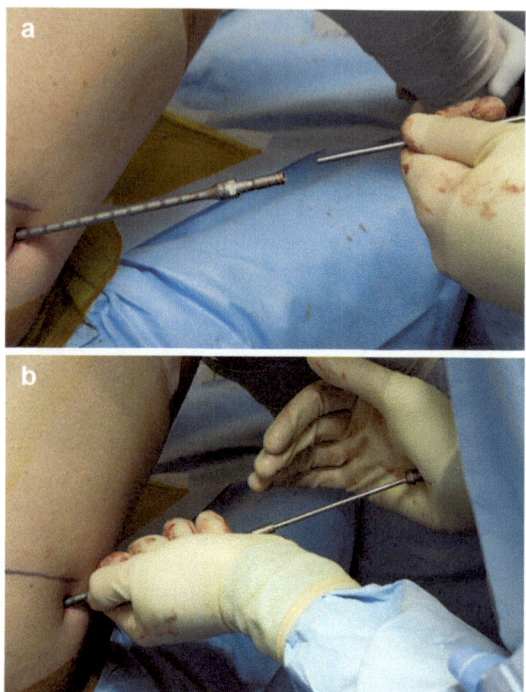

FIGURE 6.6 In order to prevent backflow of the concentrated bone marrow, a tamp (**a**) is inserted into the PerFuse cannula (Biomet Biologics), and cancellous allograft is impacted (**b**) into the trochar path

and reinserted at a different angle to push cancellous bone into the tract. Alternatively, the surgeon can choose to retract the trochar until it is out of the lesion and inject demineralized bone matrix (DBX) to plug the tract. In that case, using the plunger that comes with the system is very helpful in order to push the DBX into a superior and medial position (Fig. 6.6).

Postoperative Care

All patients are discharged home the day of surgery. Since we use a smaller trochar than is typically used for core decompression, patients are allowed to weight bearing as tolerated immediately postoperatively with the use of crutches for approximately 2 weeks. In our experience, many patients only use the crutches for less than a week. In patients such as the one in this case who undergo bilateral procedures, we recommend the use of crutches until the patient no longer has pain. A majority of patients have significant pain relief within a few weeks following the procedure; however in some patients, we have noticed an increase in pain which typically resolved by 3 months postoperative. We discharge all patients on 10 mg of simvastatin daily until healing or collapse of the lesion occurs [2, 3]. There is no range of motion restrictions following this procedure.

Outcome

The patient was contacted at the 2-week postoperative point and noted a significant reduction in her pain. She was seen back in clinic at 2 months postoperative and had no pain and healed surgical incisions. At this point, she had returned to work and performed activities as tolerated.

She was seen at 1 year postoperative and at that she continued to have pain-free hips. She had returned to her daily activities and no restrictions. Her Harris Hip Score improved to 100, and she felt her hips were "much better" than before the procedure. On MRI, there was noted to be an interval healing of the ON, with decrease in the size of the lesion as well as a decrease in the T1 hypointensity (Fig. 6.7).

Literature Review

Augmentation of femoral head decompression with concentrated iliac crest bone marrow was first described in 2002 by Hernigou et al., and in this study, the authors noted success in prevention of disease progression and pain control in patients with precollapse ON [4]. In a retrospective review of 189 hips, the authors noted a 94% success rate (prevention of total hip arthroplasty) in patients with precollapse ON, compared to only 43% success in patients with femoral head collapse [4]. Following the publication of this series, there were multiple

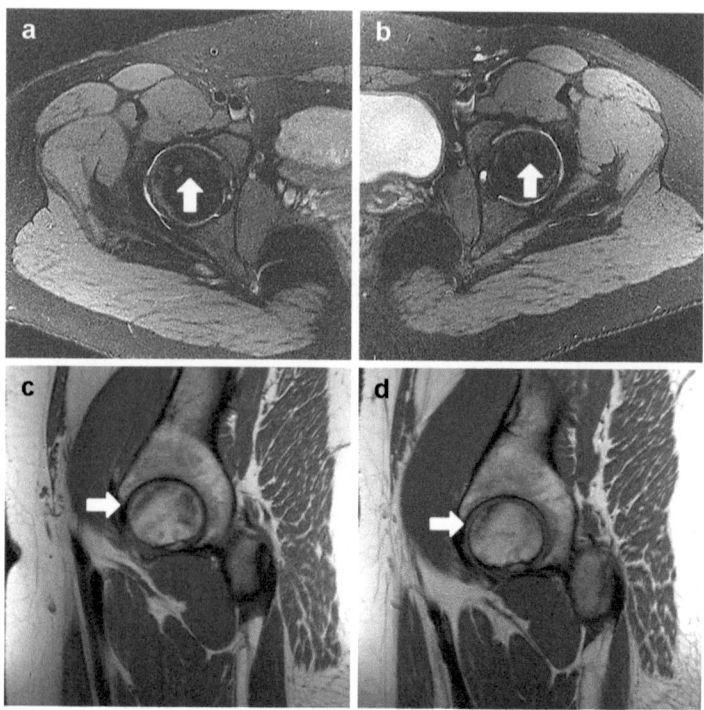

FIGURE 6.7 One year following the surgical procedure, the patient returned to clinic with resolution of the pain. On MRI there was noted to be a decrease in the size of the lesions in both hips on axial (**a, b**) as well as sagittal (**c, d**) images

prospective randomized and retrospective studies comparing core decompression to decompression augmented with MSCs (Table 6.1). With the augmentation of concentrated bone marrow to the hip decompression, up to 100% at short-term follow-up and 94% of patients at longer follow-up were able to avoid THA [4–8].

TABLE 6.1 Use of concentrated bone marrow aspirate and core decompression for the treatment of osteonecrosis of the femoral head

Study	Number of hips	Stage	Mean follow-up	Hip survival
Hernigou et al. (2002) [2]	189	Precollapse: 145 Collapse: 44	7 years	Precollapse: 94% Collapse: 43%
Gangi et al. (2004) [3]	10	Precollapse: 10	2 years	100%
Gangi et al. (2011) [4]	13	Precollapse: 13	5 years	77%
Martin et al. (2013) [7]	73	Precollapse: 73	17 months	79%
Sen et al. (2013) [5]	26	Precollapse: 26	24 months	91% (no differentiation of groups)
Rastogi et al. (2013) [6]	60	Precollapse: 60	24 months	100% with concentrated mononuclear cells 90% with bone marrow

At our institution, we have published our experience using concentrated bone marrow with platelet-rich plasma and core decompression [9]. In our use of this procedure, 86% of patients were noted to have significant pain relief. Although a majority of patients were noted to have significant pain relief, hip preservation occurred in 79% of patients at a mean of 17 months postoperative [9]. In addition to these patients progressing, additional complications included re-decompression of the femoral head with concentrated bone marrow injection in four patients and trochanteric bursitis in two patients.

We feel that further investigation into the concentrated bone marrow is needed to determine if inherent defects in the mesenchymal stem cells from patients with osteonecrosis could account for these failures [10]. Recently an in vitro study of stem cells isolated from alternative sources, such as adipose, could potentially improve outcome following this procedure, although this has yet to be shown clinically [11]. Likewise another in vitro study has shown that stem cells isolated from patients with osteonecrosis of the femoral head may have an inability to produce bone, which again could account for some of these failures [10].

Clinical Pearls and Pitfalls

- This procedure should not be used in patients where the femoral head has already collapsed.
- Start the trochar above the lesser trochanter, in order to decrease risk of subtrochanteric fracture.
- Slowly advance the trochar in order to ensure you do not penetrate the subchondral bone with the trochar during the decompression.
- If resistance is met at the time of injection, retract the trochar slowly and confirm repositioning on fluoroscopy and then inject.

References

1. Harris WH. Traumatic arthritis of the hip after dislocation and acetabular fractures: treatment by mold arthroplasty. An end-result study using a new method of result evaluation. J Bone Joint Surg Am. 1969;51(4):737–55.

2. Pritchett JW. Statin therapy decreases the risk of osteonecrosis in patients receiving steroids. Clin Orthop Relat Res. 2001;386:173–8.

3. Bowers JR, et al. Drug therapy increases bone density in osteonecrosis of the femoral head in canines. J Surg Orthop Adv. 2004;13(4):210–6.

4. Hernigou P, Beaujean F. Treatment of osteonecrosis with autologous bone marrow grafting. Clin Orthop Relat Res. 2002;405:14–23.

5. Gangji V, et al. Treatment of osteonecrosis of the femoral head with implantation of autologous bone-marrow cells. A pilot study. J Bone Joint Surg Am. 2004;86-A(6):1153–60.

6. Gangji V, De Maertelaer V, Hauzeur JP. Autologous bone marrow cell implantation in the treatment of non-traumatic osteonecrosis of the femoral head: five year follow-up of a prospective controlled study. Bone. 2011;49(5):1005–9.

7. Sen RK, et al. Early results of core decompression and autologous bone marrow mononuclear cells instillation in femoral head osteonecrosis: a randomized control study. J Arthroplasty. 2012;27(5):679–86.

8. Rastogi S, et al. Intralesional autologous mesenchymal stem cells in management of osteonecrosis of femur: a preliminary study. Musculoskelet Surg. 2013;97(3):223–8.

9. Martin JR, Houdek MT, Sierra RJ. Use of concentrated bone marrow aspirate and platelet rich plasma during minimally invasive decompression of the femoral head in the treatment of osteonecrosis. Croat Med J. 2013;54(3):219–24.

10. Houdek MT, et al. Decreased osteogenic activity of mesenchymal stem cells in patients with corticosteroid-induced osteonecrosis of the femoral head. J Arthroplasty. 2015;31:893–8.

11. Wyles CC, et al. Adipose-derived mesenchymal stem cells are phenotypically superior for regeneration in the setting of osteonecrosis of the femoral head. Clin Orthop Relat Res. 2015;473:3080–90.

Chapter 7
Core Decompression and Bone Marrow Stem Cell Injection

Hamed Vahedi and Javad Parvizi

Case Presentation

A 32-year-old female has been referred because of right hip pain. The patient has been having pain in the right groin for the past 5 months. She had, on numerous occasions, received systemic steroids for treatment of asthma. The pain is described as severe and radiates down the anteromedial thigh. The patient's level of disability necessitates using a cane to walk. She had no other pertinent medical history.

H. Vahedi, MD
Rothman Institute at Thomas Jefferson University, Philadelphia, PA, USA

J. Parvizi, MD, FRCS (✉)
James Edwards Professor of Orthopaedic Surgery, Sidney Kimmel School of Medicine, Rothman Institute at Thomas Jefferson University, Sheridan Building, Suite 1000, 125 S 9th Street, Philadelphia, PA 19107, USA
e-mail: parvj@aol.com

R.J. Sierra (ed.), *Osteonecrosis of the Femoral Head*,
DOI 10.1007/978-3-319-50664-7_7,
© Mayo Foundation for Medical Education and Research 2017

67

Diagnosis/Assessment

On physical examination, she had discomfort in the right hip at extremes of flexion, extension, abduction, adduction, and rotation.

Hip range of motion was 100° of flexion, 30° of internal rotation, and 40° of external rotation.

Radiographs and the MRI (Figs. 7.1, 7.2, and 7.3) reveal evidence of osteonecrosis of the femoral head that involves the anterolateral region with no signs of collapse (stage 2 Ficat). The joint space is normal and there is no joint effusion.

Management

Based on the presentation, physical examination and other available metrics possibility of core decompression and bone marrow injection were discussed with the patient (Fig. 7.4). The patient decided to undergo the procedure.

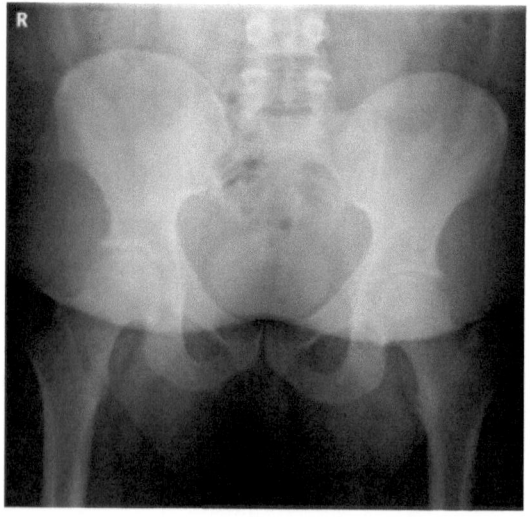

FIGURE 7.1 Pelvic AP X-ray showing *right* femoral head avascular necrosis with good joint space and no signs of collapse or flattening

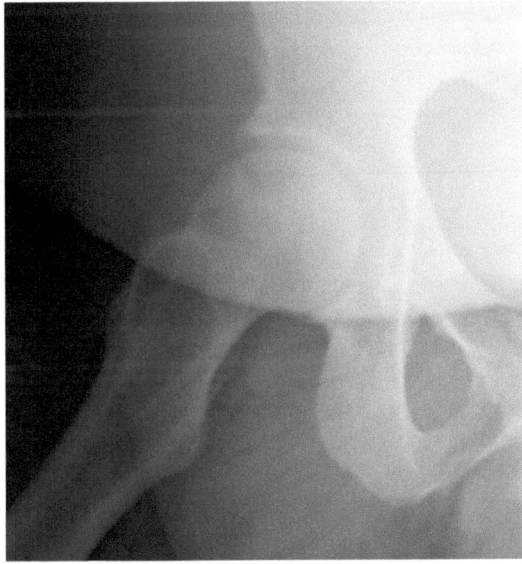

FIGURE 7.2 Hip lateral X-ray shows anterolateral lesion

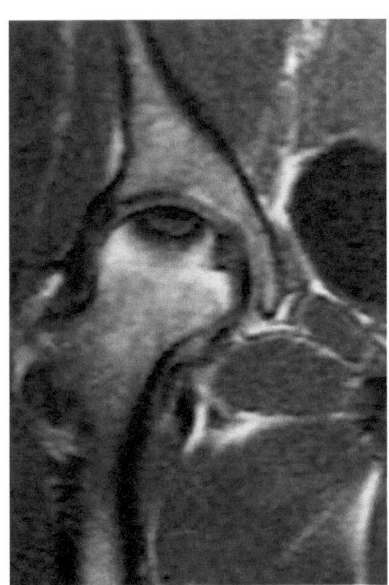

FIGURE 7.3 *Right* hip MRI shows the lesion border and extension and no signs of joint destruction or collapse of femoral head

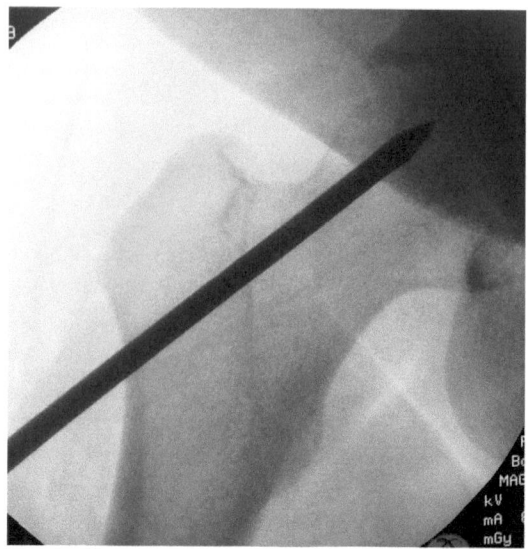

FIGURE 7.4 Core decompression using special cannulated device that was advanced into the lesion through which the bone marrow stem cells as well as platelet-rich plasma was injected

Surgical Technique and Sample Processing

Stem cells are obtained by bone marrow aspiration of the iliac crest. The marrow material from the iliac crest can be obtained percutaneously using a large-bore needle (14 gauge) advanced between the cortical tables of the crest. Approximately 120 ml of bone marrow aspirate is obtained. The bone marrow aspirate retrieved can either be processed in the operating room to obtain marrow concentrate containing stem cells or sent for expansion in the bone marrow transplant unit. We utilize both methods at our institution with preference given to expansion of the aspirate to increase the number of stems cells and better characterize them prior to injection. If expansion of the aspirate is intended, it is important to ensure that a sterile container containing cell anticoagulant solution (citric acid, sodium citrate, dextrose) is utilized to transport the aspirate. The aspirated bone marrow must be filtered and washed to remove fat, clot debris, and red blood cells (RBCs). The bone marrow is then centrifuged for 5–10 min at 400 g. To remove the heavier polynuclear cells from the periphery at a flow rate of 100 ml/min for about 50 s, the lighter anucleated RBCs and plasma are collected from the center.

All these procedures should be done under sterile conditions. After separating mononuclear cells (MNC) containing stem cells, cell count is performed. If the mean MNC count per ml is at least 2 million cells, the concentrated MNCs are then sent back to the operating room in a sterile plastic bag containing anticoagulants for injection. The processing of the bone marrow aspirate can occur in less than 60 min. We perform core decompression using the classic technique. After the preparation of the skin, a small incision is made on the lateral aspect of the hip, just below the greater trochanter. A 2.7 mm drill is advanced into the neck through the lateral cortex. The drill is advanced under fluoroscopy until it reaches the necrotic area of the femoral head. The drill is then retracted, and a spinal needle is advanced in the track of the previous drill into the femoral head to within 2–3 mm of the joint line. The expanded bone marrow material is then injected into the lesion slowly, and once complete, the needle is withdrawn. The entrance of the needle is then closed with an allograft bone plug obtained from the lateral cortex or the iliac crest.

Patients are instructed to refrain from full weight bearing for 4–6 weeks. If the patient has a bilateral surgery, a four-point gait with two crutches is encouraged. The patient is also instructed to refrain from engaging in high-impact activities for at least 6 months also.

Outcome

The core decompression and the bone marrow concentrate injection provided a considerable degree of pain relief to the patient.

Literature Review

Implanting bone marrow cells combined with core decompression for ONFH was proposed by Hernigou et al. in 2000 [1]. Subsequently some investigators have reported on their experience with stem cell therapy for osteonecrosis [2–4]. Ganji et al. [2] in a small series noted the progression of the disease in patients who received core decompression alone versus those who underwent core decompression combined with stem cell injection. This was consistent with the MRI findings of a study from our center also showing that the disease did not progress in patients who received core decompression combined with stem cell injection versus those who received core decompression alone [5]. In fact, three patients in the stem cell injection group witnessed marked improvement in their symptoms as well as the MRI appearance. Two patients had an improvement from stage 3–2, and another patient improved from stage 2–1. In contrast, ten patients in the core decompression-alone group had a deterioration of their symptoms and the MRI appearance, of whom three patients required subsequent conversion to THA. Interestingly, two patients with ARCO stage 3 who received stem cell injection also noted a marked improvement in their condition and the MRI appearance [5].

In the same study, there was a marked improvement in the functional status of the patients as measured by Western Ontario and McMaster University Osteoarthritis Index (WOMAC) questionnaire and the visual analogue scale (VAS) pain index [5]. The mean WOMAC and VAS scores in all patients improved significantly with the most marked improvement being in the group of patients that received bone marrow transplant [5].

Clinical Pearls and Pitfalls

- We advocate the use of bone marrow-derived stem cells obtained from the iliac crest as an adjuvant to core decompression for stage I and II and possibly stage III ONFH in very young patients.

References

1. Hernigou P, Habibi A, Bachir D, et al. The natural history of asymptomatic osteonecrosis of the femoral head in adults with sickle cell disease. J Bone Joint Surg Am. 2006;88-12:2565.
2. Gangji V, Hauzeur JP. Treatment of osteonecrosis of femoral head with implantation of autologous bone marrow cells. J Bone Joint Surg (Am Vol). 2005;87:10.
3. Yan ZQ, Chen YS, Li WJ, et al. Treatment of osteonecrosis of the femoral head by percutaneous decompression and autologous bone marrow mononuclear cell infusion. Chin J Traumatol. 2006;9:3.
4. Daltro GC, Fortuna VA, Salvino de Araujo SA, et al. Femoral head necrosis treatment with autologous stem cells in sickle cell disease. Acta Orthop Bras. 2008;16:44.
5. Tabatabaee RM, Sabri S, Parvizi J, et al. Combining concentrated autologous bone marrow stem cell injection with core decompression improves outcome for patients with early-stage osteonecrosis of femoral head: a comparative study. J Arthroplasty. 2015;30:11.

Chapter 8
Osteonecrosis of the Femoral Head

William C. Pannell and Jay R. Lieberman

Case Presentation
The patient was a 29-year-old male with a 1-year history of deep right buttock pain. He primarily had pain at rest that improved with activity. He denied any back pain or radiating pain. He denied any past medical or surgical history and did not take any medications regularly. The patient's major risk factor for osteonecrosis was steroid use secondary to an allergic reaction to peanuts, which happened approximately 18 months prior to the start of his symptoms. The other risk factor was the consumption of 15 alcohol drinks per week. The patient worked as a mechanical engineer.

W.C. Pannell, MD
Orthopaedic Resident, Department of Orthopaedic Surgery, Keck School of Medicine of USC, Los Angeles, CA, USA

J.R. Lieberman, MD (✉)
Department of Orthopaedic Surgery, Keck School of Medicine of USC, Los Angeles, CA, USA

Biomedical Engineering, Viterbi School of Engineering of USC, Los Angeles, CA, USA
e-mail: jrlieber@usc.edu

R.J. Sierra (ed.), *Osteonecrosis of the Femoral Head*,
DOI 10.1007/978-3-319-50664-7_8,
© Mayo Foundation for Medical Education and Research 2017

On physical examination, the patient stood 5 feet 10 inches tall and weighed 181 pounds. He walked with a normal gait. His right hip had 0–120° of flexion, 40° of external rotation, 30° internal rotation, and 40° of abduction. There was no pain with range of motion of the hip. His left hip had 0–115° of flexion, 40° of external rotation, 35° of internal rotation, and 40° of abduction. Both legs were neurovascularly intact.

Plain radiographs of the right hip showed sclerosis of the femoral head without collapse (Fig. 8.1). Preoperative MRI of the right hip showed a low intensity region in the femoral head on T1-weighted images (Fig. 8.2). At that time the patient had persistent pain and was interested in pursuing surgical management for his right hip osteonecrosis.

Diagnosis/Assessment

The patient's history, physical, and imaging were consistent with a diagnosis of osteonecrosis of the right femoral head with an atypical pain presentation. The patient's major risk factor for osteonecrosis of the hip was the prior use of steroids. Sclerosis of the femoral head without subchondral collapse on plain films, along with marrow edema on MRI, was consistent with Ficat/Steinberg stage II osteonecrosis.

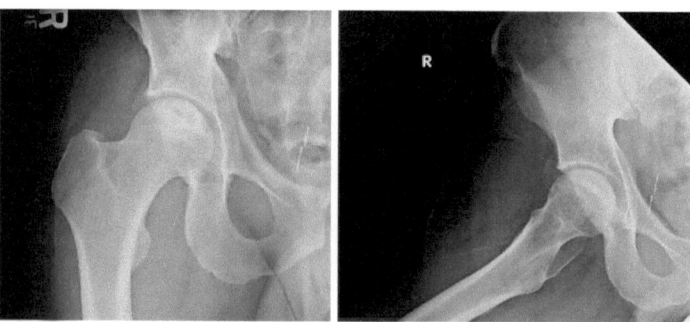

FIGURE 8.1 Preoperative anteroposterior (**a**) and lateral (**b**) radiographs of the *right* hip

FIGURE 8.2 Preoperative coronal T1-weighted MRI of the *right* hip

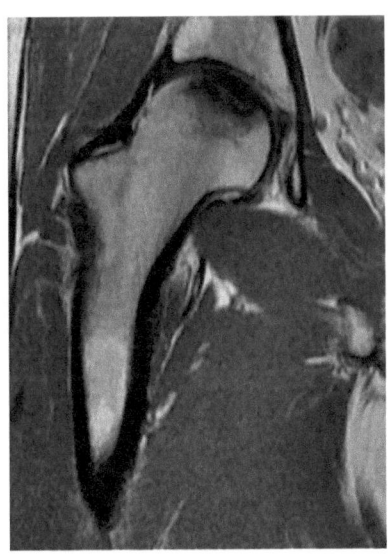

Early diagnosis of osteonecrosis of the femoral head is important to improve treatment outcomes. Patients most commonly present with deep groin pain or ipsilateral buttock pain. The patients often complain of a constant dull aching in the hip that may increase in intensity with activity or ambulation. On physical examination, range of motion may be variable. Patients may present with normal range of motion or with minimal loss of internal rotation secondary to inflammation of the joint. These findings suggest that the hip has not collapsed. A significant loss of internal rotation suggests collapse of the femoral head. A definitive diagnosis of osteonecrosis is usually made with MRI. On plain radiographs sclerosis of the femoral head is suggestive of osteonecrosis. Radiographic progression of the disease usually involves the presence of a crescent sign or frank collapse of the femoral head. The frog lateral view is the optimal view to determine the presence of a crescent sign or collapse of the femoral head. Over time the femoral head may flatten, and finally the joint space narrows and advanced degenerative changes develop. MRI is highly sensitive and specific for diagnosing osteonecrosis. T1-weighted images demonstrate a low signal intensity region representing the necrotic area. The corresponding T2-weighted images show high signal intensity because the osteonecrotic region may be surrounded by bone marrow edema. In a hip that has not collapsed, the prognosis is determined by the extent of involvement of the weight-bearing surface of the femoral head and the overall involvement of the femoral head, which can be estimated on the MRI.

Treatment of osteonecrosis of the femoral head is dependent on the severity at the time of diagnosis. Nonsurgical management has a very limited role, except in the follow-up of small and asymptomatic lesions. Biophysical and pharmacologic treatments including extracorporeal shock wave and bisphosphonates may have some role in osteonecrosis prior to collapse, although strong evidence is lacking. In a randomized controlled trial evaluating zoledronate, a bisphosphonate, patients were randomized to receive 5 mg of zoledronate or a placebo annually. The rate of total hip arthroplasty in the zoledronate group was 19 of 55 patients (35%) and in the control group was 20 of 55 (36%) at 2-year follow-up. Further randomized studies are still needed to determine if pharmacologic treatment is beneficial in early-stage disease (pre-collapse hip).

Surgical management is dependent on whether collapse of the femoral head has occurred. Prior to femoral head collapse, core decompression has been shown to be a successful treatment option. Core decompression may be performed in a number of different ways including a core tract alone, multiple small core tracts, or core decompression with bone grafting with a nonvascularized or vascularized graft or local bone grafting. Nonvascularized grafts include concentrated stem cells, demineralized bone matrix, fibular allograft, tibial allograft, and bone morphogenetic protein. Vascularized grafts are typically done with the fibula, but iliac crest grafts have also been utilized. Vascularized bone grafting, which provides both structural support and osteogenic bone graft, has also shown good long-term outcomes in patients with early-stage disease without femoral head collapse. Although these grafts have shown promise, randomized controlled trials are needed to determine if true benefits exist.

Tantalum rod insertion after decompression has not been compared in randomized trials to core decompression alone, and prospective studies have shown poor results with failure rates as high as 15% at 1 year. Tantalum rods are thought to promote bone ingrowth; however, a histopathologic analysis found that on explant of tantalum rods after 1 year, there was minimal bone ingrowth in the osteonecrotic region. A randomized controlled trial compared patients who received core decompression and tantalum rod insertion. The intervention group received a tantalum rod and targeted intra-arterial peripheral blood stem cells treated with granulocyte colony-stimulating factor (G-CSF). There were lower rates of conversion to total hip arthroplasty at the 3-year follow-up in the combination therapy group. Finally, prior to femoral head collapse, rotational osteotomies aim to transpose the osteonecrotic area from a weight-bearing to non-weight-bearing surface. Rotational osteotomies can be successful in patients with a combined necrotic angle <200° and with careful planning. However, these are technically difficult procedures. No randomized studies have been performed evaluating rotational osteotomies, and more evidence is needed to determine efficacy. Once femoral head collapse is present, or in patients with large osteonecrotic lesions, hip resurfacing arthroplasty and total hip arthroplasty are the two available treatments. Advantages of hip resurfacing arthroplasty are preservation of femoral bone stock, low dislocation rate, and rapid recovery from surgery. Disadvantages include a lack of modularity compared to THA, risk of periprosthetic fracture, and increased metal ion levels. Total hip arthroplasty is the most reliable treatment to achieve pain relief and function. Multiple studies with long-term follow-up have found high implant survival rates as well as high functional outcome scores.

Management

Core Decompression with Concentrated Stem Cell Therapy

A stab incision was made over the iliac crest and blunt dissection was carried down to bone. A trochar-type needle was inserted into the iliac crest, and 60 cc of fluid was aspirated, rotating the needle every 5 ml and changing the position of the needle every 10 ml. This technique was used to maximize bone marrow harvest and limit aspiration of blood [1]. The aspirate was placed in a centrifuge and spun, separating red blood cells in the bottom layer, mononuclear cells in the middle layer, and plasma in the top layer. The mononuclear cell layer was then filtered using a commercially available kit. The core decompression was then performed. This procedure involves debridement of necrotic bone and implantation of concentrated stem cells with biologic bone repair potential. To address the hip, a direct lateral incision was performed and dissection carried down through the skin, subcutaneous tissue, and iliotibial band. The posterior edge of the vastus lateralis fascia was incised, and the muscle was elevated off of the intermuscular septum until the underlying proximal lateral femur was identified. A radiolucent retractor was then placed to provide deep visualization of the bone. Under fluoroscopic guidance a wire was placed through the lateral aspect of the femur, across the femoral neck, and into the femoral head. The position of the guidewire was confirmed on AP and lateral fluoroscopic views. The core tract was created using ACL reamers. We started with an 8 mm reamer and reamed up to 11 mm. The diameter of the reamer used depends on the size of the femur. A burr was used to remove necrotic bone from the femoral head under fluoroscopic guidance. Additionally, a 10 mm reamer was used to create another channel just inferior to the original to allow for increased debridement of necrotic bone. Again, all reaming was performed under fluoroscopic guidance with care taken not to violate the subchondral bone.

The bone from the greater trochanter was packed into the femoral head, and then concentrated bone marrow stem cells were injected into the femoral head. The core tract was sealed using demineralized bone matrix. AP and frog lateral fluoroscopic views were obtained to confirm graft placement. The wound was irrigated and closed in the typical fashion. Postoperatively, the patient was allowed to ambulate with ten-pound flatfoot weight bearing on the operated leg using crutches for 6 weeks. Over the next 6 weeks, the weight-bearing status was advanced to weight bearing as tolerated with crutches.

In summary, the patient presented in this case with osteonecrosis of his right femoral head without collapse of the femoral head. The following management was performed: (1) aspiration of the bone marrow from the iliac crest with concentration of stem cells, (2) core decompression and core debridement of the femoral head, and (3) bone grafting of the core tract with the bone from the greater trochanter and marrow aspirate from the iliac crest with concentrated stem cells.

Outcome

This 29-year-old gentleman with bilateral femoral head osteonecrosis is now 30 months status post right hip core decompression with concentrated stem cells. He is doing well and has no pain in his groin or buttock. There is still some sclerosis in his right femoral head, but no evidence of collapse (Fig. 8.3).

Literature Review

Although numerous risk factors for osteonecrosis of the femoral head have been identified, including corticosteroid use, alcohol, trauma, and hypercoagulable states, the etiology of the disease is still unclear (Table 8.1) [2]. Ischemia of the

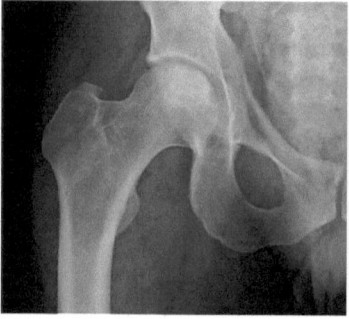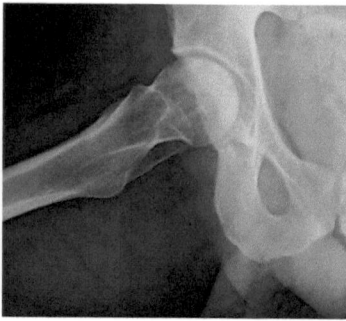

FIGURE 8.3 28-month postoperative anteroposterior (**a**) and lateral (**b**) radiographs of the *right* hip

TABLE 8.1 Risk factors for osteonecrosis

Risk factors for osteonecrosis
Corticosteroid use
Excessive alcohol consumption
Trauma
Hypercoagulable states
Smoking
Autoimmune diseases
Hyperlipidemia

femoral head through vascular disruption, constriction, or thrombosis and direct cellular toxicity likely play a role, although neither completely explains the pathogenesis of the disease [3]. A multifactorial process is certainly at play, and although risk factors have been identified, these also cannot predict who will develop the disease [4]. Surgical management is generally the recommended treatment, although nonoperative management has been studied. Bisphosphonates have been assessed as a possible treatment to prevent femoral head collapse. The hypothesis for the use of bisphosphonates is that by inhibiting osteoclast activity, and thereby blocking bone resorption, more bone formation may occur, which theoretically creates structural support in the weakened necrotic area. Chen et al. performed a multicenter randomized controlled trial comparing 65 hips (52 patients) with pre-collapse (45 hips) as well as subchondral collapse (20 hips) osteonecrosis [5]. Patients were randomized to receive either 70 mg oral alendronate or placebo weekly for 104 weeks. At 2-year follow-up, 4 (12.5%) hips in the alendronate group and 5 (15.2%) hips in the placebo group underwent THA. Lai et al. also evaluated alendronate in a randomized controlled trial of patients with pre-collapse (30 hips) and subchondral collapse (24 hips) osteonecrosis [6]. Patients were randomized to receive either 70 mg oral alendronate (29 hips) or placebo (25 hips) weekly for 25 weeks. At 2-year follow-up, one hip (3.4%) in the alendronate group and 16 hips (65%) in the control group had undergone THA ($P < 0.001$). Lee et al. performed a prospective randomized study (110 patients) to assess the efficacy of zoledronate for the management of medium to large osteonecrotic areas (>30%) without femoral head collapse [7]. Patients received either intravenous zoledronate (55 patients) or placebo (55 patients) and were followed for 2 years. The rate of total hip arthroplasty in the zoledronate group was 19 of 55 patients (35%) and in the control group was 20 of 55 (36%) at 2-year follow-up ($P = 0.796$). Zoledronate alone was also not effective in reducing the rate of collapse ($P = 0.251$).

Enoxaparin is another pharmacologic agent that has been investigated and is thought to improve blood flow to the femoral head. Glueck et al. prospectively compared 25 hips in 16 patients with thrombophilic disorders and pre-collapse femoral head osteonecrosis [8]. Nineteen of 20 hips with primary osteonecrosis did not progress radiographically at 2-year follow-up. These results suggest a potential role for etiologic-based treatment modalities. Appropriately powered randomized trials need to be performed to assess the efficacy of pharmacologic treatment alone or in combination with core decompression with bone grafting.

Core decompression is the most widely used surgical treatment to manage osteonecrosis of the femoral head without collapse and has shown promising results. A systematic review by Marker et al. found that in the last two decades 70% of patients treated with core decompression did not require additional surgery [9]. Core decompression is often supplemented with bone graft, stem cells, or biologic adjuvants to provide structural support of the osteonecrotic lesion and to promote bone formation and repair. However, this treatment regimen has not been rigorously assessed in multicenter randomized trials. Israelite et al. performed core decompression with bone grafting in 276 hips (193 patients) with a minimum 2-year follow-up [10]. In this retrospective study, the authors found that 104 hips (38%) required THA and that in patients with pre-collapse disease and small lesions, only 14% required THA. Lieberman et al. evaluated 17 hips (15 patients) treated with core decompression and the allogeneic, antigen-extracted, autolyzed cortical bone from fibular allografts combined with human bone morphogenetic protein and noncollagenous proteins. At an average follow-up of 53 months, they found that 14 hips (86%) did not have radiographic progression of osteonecrosis or conversion to THA [11]. Hernigou et al. reviewed 189 hips (116 patients) with early-stage disease treated with core decompression and autologous iliac crest bone marrow grafting [12]. The authors found that at 5-year follow-up, the total hip arthroplasty rate was 6% in patients without femoral head collapse, compared to 57% in those with femoral head collapse. In patients with early-stage disease, 103 of 136 hips (76%) did not have radiographic progression of disease, and Harris hip scores rose 17 points postoperatively. Although augmentation of core decompression with osteogenic graft or adjuvants has shown promising results, no randomized trials have been performed and are needed to determine efficacy. Lieberman et al. also recently performed a systematic review looking at operative treatment of femoral head osteonecrosis [13]. The size of the osteonecrotic lesion was found to be an important predictor of failure, and the authors found failure rates ranging from

14% to 25% after core decompression with or without grafting in patients with small lesions. Additionally, the failure rate dropped to 4.5% in cases with lesions occupying <30% of the medial weight-bearing surface. Randomized trials are needed to determine the optimal method for core decompression and whether or not biologic adjuvants improve the results.

Vascularized bone grafting can also be combined with core decompression with long-term hip survival rates between 60% and 89%, depending on the size of the necrotic region [14, 15]. Plakseychuk et al. compared vascularized to nonvascularized fibular autograft in 220 hips and found a 7-year survival rate in early-stage disease of 86% in the vascularized cohort compared to 30% in the nonvascularized group [16]. Yoo et al. reported on 14-year survival in 124 hips and found only 11% underwent total hip arthroplasty [14]. Vascularized fibular grafting has also been studied in the femoral heads that have collapsed without signs of arthrosis. Berend et al. reviewed 188 patients (224 hips) with an average follow-up of 5 years and found a conversion to total hip arthroplasty of 35% [17]. Although these results seem promising, vascularized fibular grafting is technically demanding due to the required microsurgery and is also associated with donor-site morbidity. Randomized trials are needed to determine if vascularized fibular grafts are superior to core decompression.

Tantalum rods have been investigated as an alternative to bone grafting after core decompression with the theory that the rod will act as a strut to prevent collapse of the femoral head. Veillete et al. found revision to total hip arthroplasty rates of 18% at 2 years and 32% at 4 years for early-stage disease [18]. Tanzer et al. performed histopathologic analysis on 15 of 17 tantalum implants that had been removed an average of 13 months after implantation during conversion to total hip arthroplasty and found residual osteonecrosis in 93% of implants and collapse of the femoral head in 60% [19]. The effect of tantalum rods on the natural progression of osteonecrosis is unclear, and high early failure rates between 8% and 15% reported in these studies question its efficacy when used without adjuvants [18, 19]. Tantalum rod insertion after core decompression may have a clinical benefit when combined with progenitor cells. Mao et al. performed a randomized trial of 55 patients (89 hips) comparing tantalum rod insertion alone (41 hips) to tantalum rod insertion with an intra-arterial injection of G-CSF (48 hips) [20]. G-CSF is a mobilizer of mesenchymal stem cells (MSC), and the authors hypothesized that this may increase bone formation in osteonecrotic femoral heads. The G-CSF group had conversion to total hip arthroplasty in only 3 (6%) patients, compared to 9 (22%) in the control group [20]. However, further studies are necessary before tantalum rods should be routinely used for the management of hip osteonecrosis. Another concern related to tantalum rod insertion is the potential generation of metal wear debris when rod excision is required during placement of a total hip arthroplasty (THA).

Rotational osteotomies are another option for early-stage disease, with the aim of transposing a healthy area of the femoral head to the weight-bearing area. Long-term followup after intertrochanteric osteotomies have reported between 76% and 93% success rates and is largely dependent on the size of the osteonecrotic region [21, 22]. However, rotational osteotomies are technically difficult, and the best results have not been reproduced in other centers.

While there are numerous operative treatments available, the best treatment of pre-collapse femoral head osteonecrosis is unclear. Lieberman et al. performed a systematic review of articles assessing different surgical treatments aimed at preserving the femoral head [13]. The authors included both prospective and retrospective studies with a minimum follow-up of 2 years. In hips that had not yet collapsed, 19% (409 of 2163) were converted to THA, and 31% (264 of 864) had radiographic progression of disease. In hips that had evidence of collapse, 30% (442 of 1463) were converted to THA, and 49% (419 of 850) had radiographic progression of disease. The authors were unable to identify an individual procedure with superior outcomes with regard to preventing THA or radiographic progression and noted that operative procedures aimed at preventing disease progression were not helpful in treating collapsed hips.

Once femoral head collapse has occurred, hip arthroplasty is recommended and has been shown to provide adequate pain relief and return of function in patients. Mont et al. published a comprehensive review of the efficacy and survivorship of total hip arthroplasty in patients with nontraumatic osteonecrosis of the femoral head [23]. The authors cite over 20 studies with the majority demonstrating greater than 95% implant survival, even with greater than 10-year follow-up. Kim et al. evaluated 64 hips in patients younger than 50 years old with minimum 15-year follow-up and found that no patients required revision of femoral stems for aseptic loosening, and Harris hip scores improved from 36 to 92.7 points [24]. Similarly, Bedard et al. evaluated 60 hips with an average age of 43 years who underwent noncemented THA and found that one patient (1.6%) had revision of their femoral component for aseptic loosening at 10-year follow-up [25]. Harris hip scores also improved from 49.5 preoperatively to 80.3 at latest follow-up. Issa et al. evaluated two cohorts of patients with osteonecrosis, one with sickle cell disease (42 hips) and one without (102 hips), and found no significant difference in outcomes between the groups [26]. Aseptic implant survival was 95% at 7.5-year follow-up in the sickle cell group and 97% at 7-year follow-up in the non-sickle cell group. Total hip arthroplasty has also shown promising results in very young patient groups. Kim et al. reviewed 127 hips (96 patients) in patients younger than 30 years old who underwent a ceramic-bearing THA with an average follow up of 14.8 years (range 10–16) follow-up [27]. No patients had revision of either femoral or acetabular components for aseptic loosening, and Harris hip scores improved from 41 to 95 points at final follow-up. Kim et al. also evaluated a cohort of patients with osteonecrosis who underwent THA with and without cement with 17-year follow-up (range 16–18 years) [28]. The authors found a femoral component survival rate of 98% in both groups and acetabular component survival rates of 83 and 85% in the cemented and cementless groups, respectively. Cementless total hip arthroplasty has shown good long-term results at greater than 10-year follow-up as a treatment for post-collapse osteonecrosis of the femoral head (Table 8.2).

Hip resurfacing arthroplasty is an alternative to total hip arthroplasty in young patients with collapse of the femoral

TABLE 8.2 Results of total hip arthroplasty for the treatment of osteonecrosis with minimum 10-year follow-up

Author	No. hips (patients)	Femoral component	Mean follow-up (range) (year)	Femoral component revision rate	Acetabular component revision rate	Mean Harris hip score (range)
Kim et al. [24]	64 (55)	Cementless	15.8 (15–16.8)	3 (4.7%)	14 (21.9%)	93 (72–100)
Bedard et al. [25]	80 (66)	Cementless	12.6 (9.1–16.4)	3 (3.8%)	0 (0%)	80 (5–100)
Han et al. [29]	95 (76)	Cementless	12.7 (10.7–17.3)	4 (4.2%)	NA	91 (66–100)
Min et al. [30]	58 (45)	Cementless	11.1 (10–13.4)	2 (3.4%)	19 (33%)	93 (82–99)
Kim et al. [27]	127 (96)	Cementless	14.8 (10–16)	0 (0%)	1 (0.8%)	95 (71–100)
Kim et al. [28]	148 (98)	Cementless[a]	17.3 (16–18)	3 (2.0%)	23 (16%)	93 (75–100)
Solarino et al. [31]	61 (55)	Cementless	12.9 (11–15)	1 (1.6%)	2 (3.2%)	91 (68–100)
Koch et al. [32]	32 (29)	Cemented	11.8 (10–15)	1 (3.1%)	0 (0%)	NR
Nich et al. [33]	122 (96)	Cemented	12.8 (10–20.9)	6 (4.9%)	7 (5.7%)	NR
Xenakis et al. [34]	36 (28)	Cementless	11.2 (10–15)	0 (0%)	2 (5.5%)	NR

[a]Fifty patients had cemented femoral components

head and good bone stock. A major concern with hip resurfacing arthroplasty is long-term fixation of the prosthesis if there is osteonecrosis present. Other issues related to hip resurfacing arthroplasty include periprosthetic femoral neck fracture and the potential development of pseudotumors secondary to the generation of metallic wear debris. In general, young males with large femoral heads and good bone stock in the femoral neck have the best results with hip resurfacing. However, the potential risks associated with the metal on metal-bearing surface must be thoroughly discussed with the patient. Amstutz et al. reviewed 85 hips (70 patients) that underwent hip resurfacing arthroplasty for osteonecrosis and assessed 915 hips (768 patients) without osteonecrosis for comparison [35]. The osteonecrosis group had 4 revisions (4.7%), and the control group had 35 (3.8%) at 8-year follow-up ($P = 0.6214$). Harris hip scores averaged 91.3 (range 42–100) in the osteonecrosis group and 93.5 (range 41–100) in the control group ($P = 0.1129$). Sayeed et al. compared 20 hips (17 patients) that underwent resurfacing arthroplasty to a matched cohort of 20 hips (16 patients) who underwent THA in patients 25 years of age or younger [36]. At 7.5-year follow-up, there was 100% survival in the resurfacing group and 93.3% (one patient) for the THA group. Harris hip scores averaged 93 points (range 75–100) and 94 points (range 86–100) for the resurfacing and THA groups, respectively. Nakasone et al. reviewed 39 hips (33 patients) that underwent hip resurfacing with a mean follow-up of 8 years and used MRI to classify patients based on the volume of osteonecrosis in the femoral head after machining [37]. There was one revision (5.6%) in a patient with lesion volume <25% and one revision (4.8%) in a patient with lesion volume >25%. It is intuitive that hips with large areas of osteonecrosis may not allow adequate interdigitation of cement in the femoral head, which could lead to early failure. An insightful commentary by Michael Mont, M.D., proposed the need for larger studies that may provide surgeons with the data to determine the influence of lesion size on outcomes of hip resurfacing [38].

Clinical Pearls and Pitfalls

- The key to the management of osteonecrosis of the femoral head is to determine which stage of the disease the patient has and to determine if the femoral head has collapsed.
- Patients with limited or no internal rotation of the hip generally have collapse of the femoral head.
- Nonoperative management is generally not indicated, with the exception of monitoring for progression of small lesions.
- Pharmacologic management, including bisphosphonates, requires further investigation.
- Prior to femoral head collapse, core decompression can be attempted with or without bone grafting of the femoral head.
- Patients with collapse of the femoral head with significant pain and disability should be treated with a total hip arthroplasty.

References

1. Muschler G, Boehm C, Easley K. Aspiration to obtain osteoblast progenitor cells from human bone marrow: the influence of aspiration volume. J Bone Joint Surg Am. 1997;79(11):1699–709.
2. Zalavras C, Lieberman JR. Osteonecrosis of the femoral head: evaluation and treatment. J Am Acad Orthop Surg. 2014;22:455–64.
3. Zalavras C, Dailiana Z, Elisaf M, et al. Potential aetiological factors concerning the development of osteonecrosis of the femoral head. Eur J Clin Invest. 2000;30(3):215–21.
4. Lieberman JR, Roth KM, Elsissy P, Dorey FJ, Kobashigawa JA. Symptomatic osteonecrosis of the hip and knee after cardiac transplantation. J Arthroplasty. 2008;23(1):90–6.
5. Chen CH, Chang JK, Lai KA, Hou SM, Chang CH, Wang GJ. Alendronate in the prevention of collapse of the femoral

head in nontraumatic osteonecrosis. Arthritis Rheum. 2012;64(5):1572–8.

6. Lai KA, Shen WJ, Yang CY, Shao CJ, Hsu JT, Lin RM. The use of alendronate to prevent early collapse of the femoral head in patients with nontraumatic osteonecrosis. J Bone Joint Surg Am. 2005;87-A(10):2155–9.

7. Lee YK, Ha YC, Cho YJ. Does zoledronate prevent femoral head collapse from osteonecrosis? A prospective, randomized, open-label, multicenter study. J Bone Joint Surg Am. 2015;97(14):1142–8.

8. Glueck C, Freiberg R, Sieve I, Wang P. Enoxaparin prevents progression of stages I and II osteonecrosis of the hip. Clin Orthop Relat Res. 2005;435:164–70.

9. Marker DR, Seyler TM, Ulrich SD, Srivastava S, Mont MA. Do modern techniques improve core decompression outcomes for hip osteonecrosis? Clin Orthop Relat Res. 2008;446(5):1093–103.

10. Israelite C, Nelson CL, Ziarani CF, Abboud JA, Landa J, Steinberg ME. Bilateral core decompression for osteonecrosis of the femoral head. Clin Orthop Relat Res. 2005;441:285–90.

11. Lieberman JR, Conduah A, Urist MR. Treatment of osteonecrosis of the femoral head with core decompression and human bone morphogenetic protein. Clin Orthop Relat Res. 2004;429:139–45.

12. Hernigou P, Beaujean F. Treatment of osteonecrosis with autologous bone marrow grafting. Clin Orthop Relat Res. 2002;405:14–23.

13. Lieberman JR, Engstrom S, Meneghini R, SooHoo N. Which factors influence preservation of the osteonecrotic femoral head? Clin Orthop Relat Res. 2012;470:5235–535.

14. Yoo MC, Kim KI, Hahn CS, Parvizi J. Long-term followup of vascularized fibular grafting for femoral head necrosis. Clin Orthop Relat Res. 2008;466(5):1133–40.

15. Edward WC, Rineer CA, Urbaniak JR, Richard MJ, Ruch DS. The vascularized fibular graft in precollapse osteonecrosis: is long-term hip preservation possible? Clin Orthop Relat Res. 2012;470(10):2819–26.

16. Plakseychuk AY, Kim SY, Park BC, Varitimidis SE, Rubash HE, Sotereanos DG. Vascularized compared with nonvascularized fibular grafting for the treatment of osteonecrosis of the femoral head. J Bone Joint Surg Am. 2003;85(4):589–96.

17. Berend K, Gunneson E, Urbaniak J, Vail T. Free vascularized fibular grafting for the treatment of postcollapse osteonecrosis of the femoral head. J Bone Joint Surg Am. 2003;85-A(6):987–93.

18. Veillete CJ, Mehdian H, Schemitsch EH, McKee MD. Survivorship analysis and radiographic outcome following tantalum rod insertion for osteonecrosis of the femoral head. J Bone Joint Surg Am. 2006;88(3):48–55.

19. Tanzer M, Bobyn JD, Krygier JJ, Karabasz D. Histopathologic retrieval analysis of clinically failed porous tantalum osteonecrosis implants. J Bone Joint Surg Am. 2008;90(6):1282–9.

20. Mao Q, Wang W, Xu T. Combination treatment of biomechanical support and targeted intra-arterial infusion of peripheral blood stem cells mobilized by granulocyte-colony stimulating factor for the osteonecrosis of the femoral head: a randomized controlled clinical trial. J Bone Miner Res. 2015;30(4):647–56.

21. Sugioka Y, Yamamoto T. Transtrochanteric posterior rotational osteotomy for osteonecrosis. Clin Orthop Relat Res. 2008;466(5): 1104–9.

22. Mont MA, Fairbank AC, Krackow KA, Hungerford DS. Corrective osteotomy for osteonecrosis of the femoral head. J Bone Joint Surg Am. 1996;78(7):1032–8.

23. Mont M, Cherian J, Sierra R, Jones L, Lieberman J. Nontraumatic osteonecrosis of the femoral head: where do we stand today? J Bone Joint Surg Am. 2015;97:604–27.

24. Kim SM, Lim SJ, Moon YW, Kim YT, Ko KR, Park YS. Cementless modular total hip arthroplasty in patients younger than fifty with femoral head osteonecrosis: minimum fifteen-year follow-up. J Arthroplasty. 2013;28(3):504–409.

25. Bedard NA, Callaghan JJ, Liu SS, Greiner JJ, Klaassen AL, Johnston RC. Cementless THA for the treatment of osteonecrosis at 10-year follow-up: have we improved compared to cemented THA? J Arthroplasty. 2013;28(7):1192–9.

26. Issa K, Naziri Q, Maheshwari A, Rasquinha V, Delanois R, Mont M. Excellent results and minimal complications of total hip arthroplasty in sickle cell hemoglobinopathy at mid-term follow-up using cementless prosthetic components. J Arthroplasty. 2013;28:1693–8.

27. Kim YH, Park JW, Kim JS. Cementless metaphyseal fitting anatomic total hip arthroplasty with a ceramic-on-ceramic bearing in patients thirty years of age or younger. J Bone Joint Surg Am. 2012;94:1570–5.

28. Kim YH, Kim JS, Park JW, Joo JH. Contemporary total hip arthroplasty with and without cement in patients with osteone-

crosis of the femoral head. J Bone Joint Surg Am. 2011;92:675–81.

29. Han S, Lee J, Kim J, Oh C, Kim S. Long-term durability of the CLS femoral prosthesis in patients with osteonecrosis of the femoral head. J Arthroplasty. 2013;28(5):828–31.

30. Min BW, Song KS, Bae KC, Cho CH, Lee KJ, Kim HJ. Second-generation cementless total hip arthroplasty in patients with osteonecrosis of the femoral head. J Arthroplasty. 2008;23(6):902–10.

31. Solarino G, Piazzolla A, Notarnicola A, Moretti L, Tafuri S, DeGiorgi S, Moretti B. Long-term results of 32-mm alumina-on-alumina THA for avascular necrosis of the femoral head. J Orthop Traumatol. 2012;13:21–7.

32. Koch P, Tannast M, Fujita H, Siebenrock K, Ganz R. Minimum ten year results of total hip arthroplasty with the acetabular reinforcement ring in avascular osteonecrosis. Int Orthop. 2008;32(2):173–9.

33. Nich C, Courpied J, Kerboull M, Postel M, Hamadouche M. Charnley-Kerboull total hip arthroplasty for osteonecrosis of the femoral head a minimal 10-year follow-up study. J Arthroplasty. 2006;21(4):533–40.

34. Xenakis T, Gelalis J, Koukoubis T, Zaharis K, Soucacos P. Cementless hip arthroplasty in the treatment of patients with femoral head necrosis. Clin Orthop Relat Res. 2001;386:93–9.

35. Amstutz HC, Le Duff MJ. Hip resurfacing results for osteonecrosis are as good as for other etiologies at 2 to 12 Years. Clin Orthop Relat Res. 2010;468:375–81.

36. Sayeed S, Johnson A, Stroh A, Gross T, Mont M. Hip resurfacing in patients who have osteonecrosis and are 25 years or under. Clin Orthop Relat Res. 2011;469:1582–8.

37. Nakasone S, Takao M, Sakai T, Nishii T, Sugano N. Does the extent of osteonecrosis affect the survival of hip resurfacing? Clin Orthop Relat Res. 2013;471:1926–34.

38. Mont M. CORR insights: does the extent of osteonecrosis affect the survival of hip resurfacing? Clin Orthop Relat Res. 2013;471:1935–6.

Chapter 9
Bilateral Hip Decompression Using X-REAM® and PRO-DENSE®

Eric M. Greber, Paul K. Edwards, and C. Lowry Barnes

Case Presentation

The patient is a 39-year-old Caucasian male construction worker who presents to clinic with bilateral hip pain. The pain in the left hip is worse than the right hip. The patient's left hip pain has recently gotten worse and is affecting him daily at work. His left hip originally became painful about 5 years ago, and within a few months, the right hip has started to hurt as well. The nature of the pain has always been dull, aching pain and is intensified by walking, bending down, and climbing stairs. He denies any radiation of the pain in either leg. The patient describes his pain as a 10/10 on pain scale at its worst but is 6/10 at rest bilaterally.

E.M. Greber, MD • P.K. Edwards, MD • C.L. Barnes, MD (✉)
Department of Orthopaedic Surgery, University of Arkansas for Medical Sciences, Little Rock, AR, USA
e-mail: clbarnes@uams.edu

R.J. Sierra (ed.), *Osteonecrosis of the Femoral Head*,
DOI 10.1007/978-3-319-50664-7_9,
© Mayo Foundation for Medical Education and Research 2017

One year ago he saw his primary care physician for the bilateral hip pain. He did have X-rays taken at that time, but he was told they were "negative." He was diagnosed with muscle pain from overuse at his job. He did have formal physical therapy for about 6 weeks. Physical therapy did not help his pain. He has been unable to take NSAIDs secondary to a past stomach ulcer.

He does not report any trauma or inciting event for the hip pain. He has never taken any medications on a regular basis, including steroids. He has no other significant medical problems. He does report drinking 3–4 alcoholic beverages every night.

On physical exam, the patient is a healthy-appearing male. He is 6'0" and weighs 210 lbs. His vital signs are within normal limits. He walks with a slight antalgic gait and seems to be favoring his left lower extremity with a decreased stance phase on the left compared to the right. His bilateral lower extremities have normal muscle strength in all muscle groups. He has no pain with straight leg raise testing. He has decreased internal rotation with approximately 15° on the left and 20° on the right. He has pain in both hips with hip flexion and internal rotation. He has normal sensation in bilateral lower extremities.

A standing AP X-ray of the pelvis and lateral X-rays of the bilateral hips (Fig. 9.1a–e) showed mild sclerosis in the femoral head bilateral but no arthritic changes of the hips. Joint space is maintained throughout. There is no obvious collapse of the articular surface of the femoral heads. MRI was then obtained and showed subcapital area of heterogeneous signal abnormality with a thin serpiginous rim of decreased of enhancement on TI with an increased intensity of signal on TI compared to rim (Fig. 9.2a–c). There are also patchy areas of high signal intensity on fat-saturated T2-weighted images in the femoral heads consistent with bilateral osteonecrosis of the femoral heads.

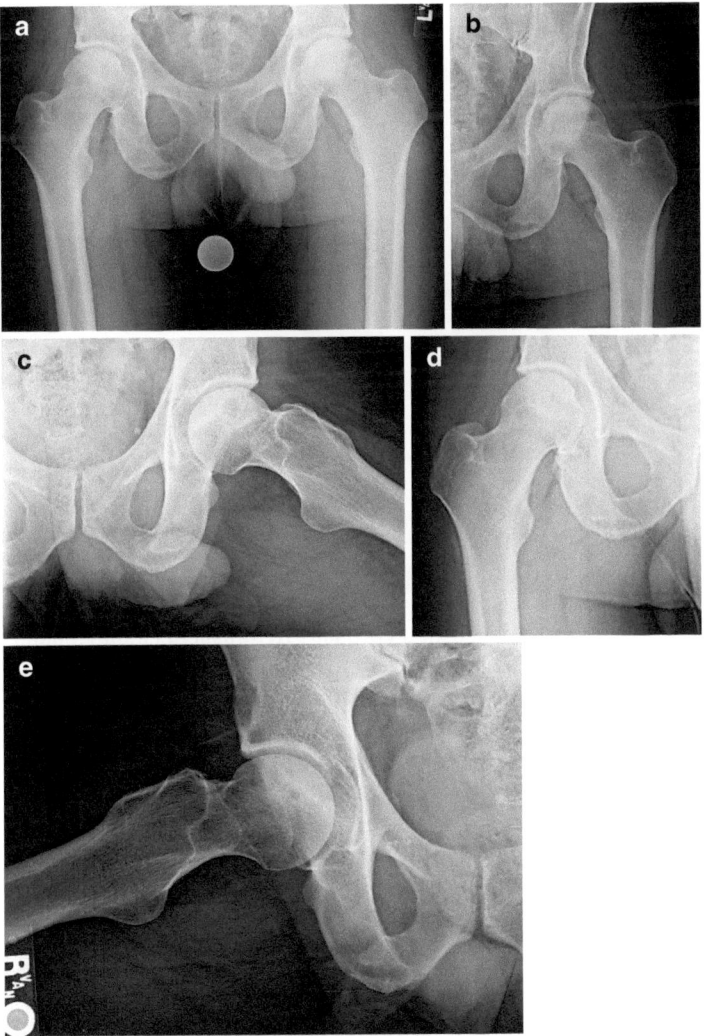

FIGURE 9.1 (**a**) Standing AP of bilateral hips. (**b**) Standing AP of the left hip. (**c**) Frog-leg lateral of the left hip. (**d**) Standing AP of the right hip. (**e**) Frog-leg lateral of the right hip

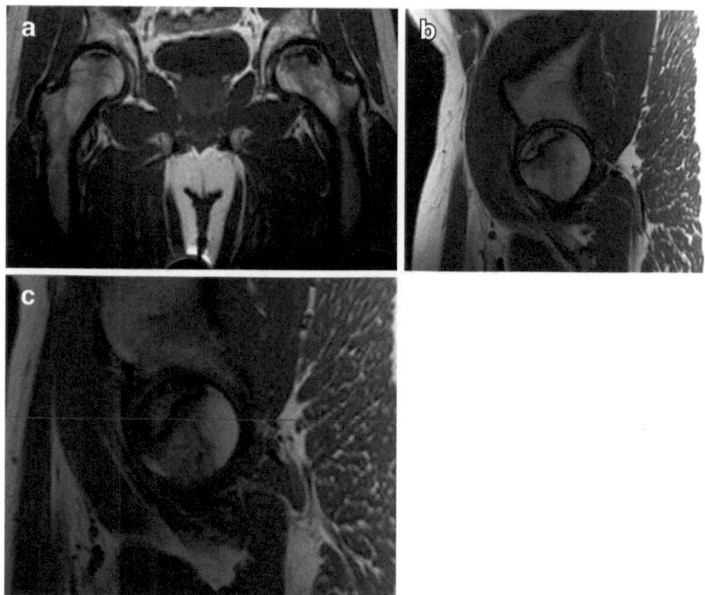

FIGURE 9.2 (a) T1-weighted coronal MRI image including bilateral hips. (b) T1-weighted sagittal MRI image of the left hip. (c) T1-weighted sagittal MRI image of the right hip

Diagnosis/Assessment

After evaluating the radiographs and MRI of this patient and comparing to history and physical exam, it is evident that he suffers from bilateral femoral head osteonecrosis. Although the etiology of the AVN in this patient is not fully understood, it can be assumed that the extensive alcohol use for long period of time is a significant risk factor. Regardless of etiology, it is unlikely that the pain in the hips will improve without intervention, but, more likely, will progress over time. Ohzono et al. reported 69% progression of Ficat stage II disease advancing to stage IV within 6 years [1]. The natural progression of larger areas of osteonecrosis of the femoral head, especially in the weight-bearing surface, includes progression to articular surface collapse secondary to the lack of structural support from the underlying affected bone. This causes the femoral head to lose its spherical congruency with the acetabulum during articulation and progresses to articular cartilage loss and arthritic changes in the hip. It is not possible at this time to predict how long this process may take in each patient.

Treatment of AVN has been a challenging issue for physicians. The mainstay of treatment for pre-collapse AVN is core decompression of the lesion. Once there is collapse of the articular surface, there is limited role for core decompression, and the surgeon may be forced to start considering arthroplasty options. The goal of treatment of early stages of AVN is to increase the blood supply to the area to stop the progression to collapse. Since this condition is common in the younger patient, it is of utmost importance that the surgeon does everything possible to achieve this lofty goal.

Our patient does not have collapse of either femoral head, and therefore the discussion of arthroplasty options for advanced AVN will not be discussed in this case report. Core decompression is a general term for an operation that has been described in many different variations. Below we will describe a technique for core decompression using an expandable reamer and calcium sulfate/calcium phosphate injectable graft.

Management

The patient was positioned supine in the operating room. Fluoroscopy was used before the case started to ensure that proper films, including AP and lateral of the femoral head, could be obtained. The instruments for X-REAM® core decompression come in a prepackaged set from the supplier (Wright Medical Technology, Memphis, TN, USA). The guidewire from the set was then placed on the anterior thigh/groin and adjusted until the tip of the guidewire is overlying the known region of AVN in the femoral head. A small 3–4 cm incision was then made on the lateral side of the thigh at the level of the femur in line with guidewire projection. The

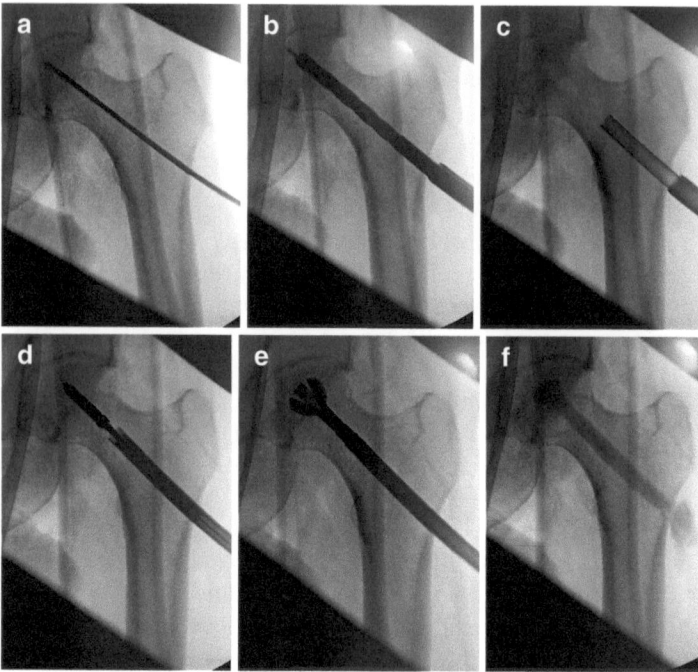

FIGURE 9.3 (**a**) 3.2 mm guidewire from X-REAM set is drilled into the area of the femoral head where the lesion is based off of preoperative planning from MRI. (**b**) 9 mm cannulated drill. (**c**) Working cannula is placed up the drill from the previous step. This cannula will be left in place to place instruments through for the rest of the procedure. (**d**) X-REAM® reamer placed through working cannula. Reamer has not been expanded yet. (**e**) Fluoroscopy of the X-REAM® in full expansion reaming the lesion in the femoral head. (**f**) PRO-DENSE® injected into the decompression tract

guidewire is then inserted into the wound and drilled into the femoral neck into the region of the AVN (Fig. 9.3a). Orthogonal views of fluoroscopy were used to ensure that the guidewire is in the area of the femoral head that was planned from the preoperative MRI. The 9 mm cannulated drill is then placed over the guidewire (Fig. 9.3b). Once removed, the working cannula which is part of the set is placed in the drill tunnel that has now been made in the femoral neck (Fig. 9.3c).

X-REAM® is an expandable reamer which is drilled into the femoral head lesion and slowly expanded by rotating the mechanism in the handle of the reamer (Fig. 9.4a, b). The expansion allows for a 2.1 cm ream in the lesion at the femoral head once fully expanded (Fig. 9.4c). The expandable reamer was placed over the guidewire into the lesion in the femoral head (Fig. 9.3d). Once to the appropriate depth confirmed by fluoroscopy, the expansion of the reamer was performed (Fig. 9.3e). This is done by turning the knob of the reamer a quarter turn at a time. The reaming is performed after each quarter turn expansion. Throughout the reaming process, it is paramount that the fluoroscopy is used to ensure that the reamer is not getting to close to the articular cartilage. After reaming with the reamer in full expansion, the knob on the back of the reamer is turned counterclockwise to retract the blades back to original position, and the reamer is then removed from the femur. At this time, through the working cannula, curettage of the lesion was performed and suctioned out using the curette and suction tip from the set.

The PRO-DENSE® synthetic bone graft is mixed on the back table and placed in the syringe. The syringe is then placed into the femur all the way to the tip of the reamed area. The entire tract of the core decompression was then injected with PRO-DENSE® (Fig. 9.3f). Care is taken to irrigate the graft that leaked out under the IT band. The wounds were then closed in a routine fashion.

Outcome

The patient was discharged from the hospital on the same day of surgery with a walker. Although he was instructed to touch down weight bear only for the first 6 weeks per our routine, he started full weight bearing on the second postoperative day. At his 2-week follow-up visit, the patient

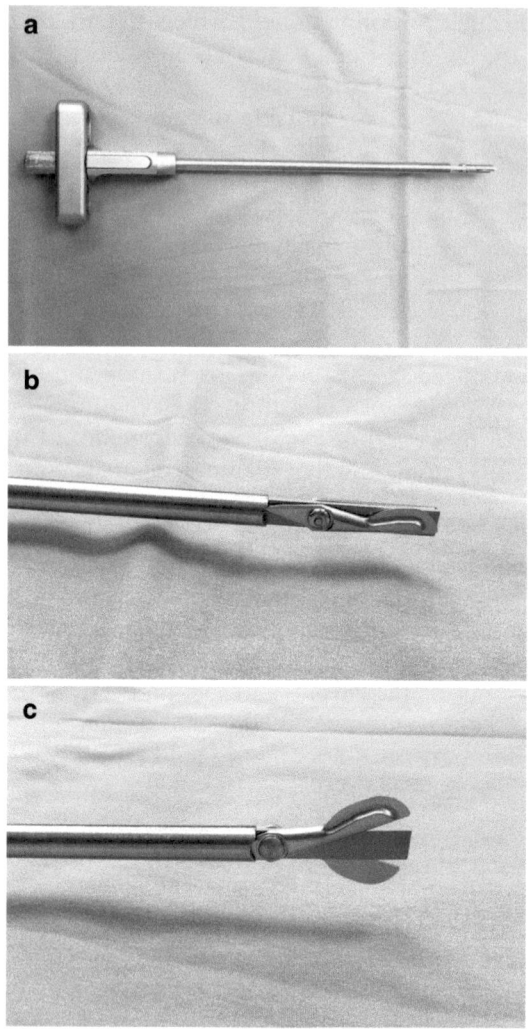

FIGURE 9.4 (**a**) X-REAM® expandable reamer (Wright Medical Technology, Memphis, TN USA) in non-expanded form. Expansion of the reamer blades is performed by rotating the threaded part of the handle on the end of the reamer. (**b**) Close-up view of non-expanded position of the X-REAM® expandable reamer. (**c**) X-REAM® reamer after expansion of the blades

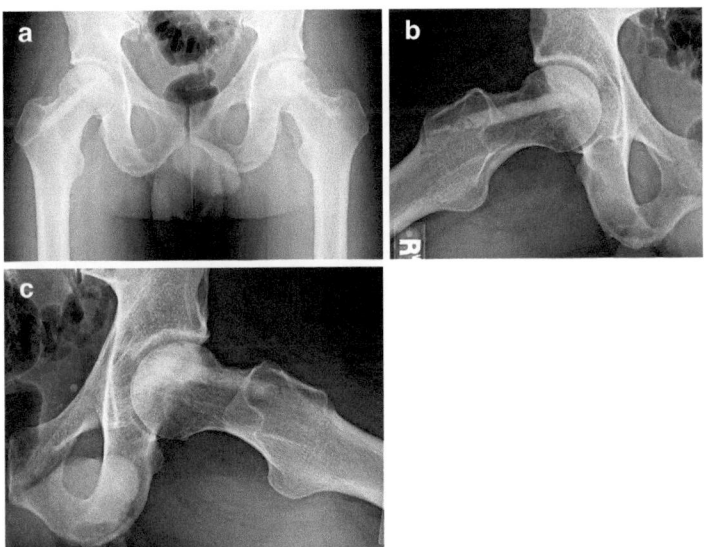

FIGURE 9.5 (**a**) Standing AP pelvis at 2 weeks postoperative follow-up visit. (**b**) Frog-leg lateral of the right hip at 2 weeks postoperative follow-up visit. (**c**) Frog-leg lateral of the left hip at 2 weeks postoperative follow-up visit

was walking without a limp for first time in approximately 6 months. Radiographs show no progression of disease (Fig. 9.5a–c). He reports no pain. At his final follow-up visit 1 year from date of surgery, he was still having no pain, and radiographs showed evidence of healing at the core decompression site. There was no sign of collapse of the femoral head at the final follow-up.

Literature Review

Although there is a significant amount literature published on treatment on AVN of the femoral head, there is a paucity of literature published on treatment of AVN with X-REAM®

expandable reamer and supplementation with PRO-DENSE® calcium sulfate/calcium phosphate. The literature shows unpredictable results with many different surgical techniques highlighting the treatment challenge that AVN of the femoral head continues to present for the orthopedic surgeon. Success rate for preventing radiographic progression of disease regardless of the surgical technique is variable in the literature with results ranging from 29 to 83% for Ficat stage I and IIA [2, 3].

The concept of using the X-REAM® system attempts to avoid weakening the femoral neck from the drill and therefore theoretically preventing postoperative femoral neck fractures. The expandable reamer used in this technique allows the surgeon to create a smaller drill in the femoral neck and simultaneously allows for larger lesion decompression in the head. The drill for the core decompression is 9 mm in diameter, and the reamer then expands to a diameter of 2.1 cm.

PRO-DENSE® is composed of calcium sulfate and calcium phosphate together in a composite graft. The graft combines the advantages of both types of synthetic grafts and is thought to have osteoconductive properties. This combination has been found in canine model studies to have increase bone formation in comparison to normal bone as well as having ultimate compression strength greater than normal bone at 13 and 26 weeks after administration. The modulus of elasticity at 13 and 26 weeks of the restored bone when the graft is used is not significantly different than normal bone [4]. There have been no trials in humans that test mechanical strength and histology of regenerated bone. Civinini et al. have published the only clinical study on this technique to our knowledge. They reported 78.4% radiographic success rate (not progression to collapse) and only 3.3% clinical failure rate in pre-collapse group defined by conversion to arthroplasty. The study mean follow-up was 20.6 months [5].

Osteonecrosis of the femoral head continues to be a challenge for the orthopedic surgeon as there are many different surgical techniques and options. Gold standard for early-stage osteonecrosis of the femoral head (Ficat I and IIA) is still considered core decompression. The X-REAM® supplemented with PRO-DENSE® composite graft continues to be the authors' preferred method of choice for core decompression.

Clinical Pearls and Pitfalls

- Like all other core decompression techniques, this is not indicated in post-collapse osteonecrosis.
- Place reamer tip in position keeping in mind the diameter of expansion (more than double the size of the ream tip unexpanded) so as not to break the subchondral bone.
- Take care when injecting the PRO-DENSE® to make sure that it does not spill out of the core decompression hole and collect under the IT band.
- Can use specific curette and suction that comes in the set to clean the lesion through the working cannula.
- Expansion of the reamer should be slow because the bone will be very hard and sclerotic and could cause failure of the expandable reamer.

References

1. Ohzono K, Saito M, Takaoka K, Ono K, Saito S, Nishina T, Kadowaki T. Natural history of nontraumatic avascular necrosis of the femoral head. J Bone Joint Surg. 1991;73-B:68–72.
2. Smith SW, Fehring TK, Griffin WL, Beaver WB. Core decompression of the osteonecrotic femoral head. J Bone Joint Surg. 1995;77-A:674–80.
3. Learmonth ID, Maloon S, Dall G. Core decompression for early atraumatic osteonecrosis of the femoral head. J Bone Joint Surg. 1990;72-B:387–90.
4. Urban RM, Turner TM, Hall DJ, Inoue N, Gitelis S. Increased bone formation using calcium sulphate-calcium phosphate composite graft. Clin Orthop Relat Res. 2007;459:110–7.
5. Civinini R, De Biase P, Carulli C, Matassi F, Nistri L, Capanna R, Innocenti M. The use of injectable calcium sulphate/calcium phosphate bioceramic in the treatment of osteonecrosis of the femoral head. Int Orthop. 2012;36:1583–8.

Chapter 10
Surgical Dislocation and Osteochondral Autograft Transfer System (OATS) as Salvage of Failed Core Decompression Complicated by Femoral Head Penetration

Cody C. Wyles and Rafael J. Sierra

Case Presentation

A 25-year-old female school teacher presented with unresolved right groin pain after core decompression performed at an outside institution 10 months prior. She had a history of renal failure in the setting of IgA nephropathy requiring several prolonged courses of corticosteroid therapy; however, this was not part of the medication regimen at the time of presentation to our facility. Outside records indicated that she was treated with right core decompression augmented with

C.C. Wyles, MD • R.J. Sierra, MD (✉)
Department of Orthopaedic Surgery, Mayo Clinic,
Rochester, MN 55905, USA
e-mail: sierra.rafael@mayo.edu

R.J. Sierra (ed.), *Osteonecrosis of the Femoral Head*,
DOI 10.1007/978-3-319-50664-7_10,
© Mayo Foundation for Medical Education and Research 2017

Pro-Dense® graft (Wright Medical Technology, Inc., Memphis, Tennessee, USA). Postoperatively, she was managed with protected weight bearing and gradual advancement of activity. She discontinued using crutches after 2 months and a cane after 3 months. Nevertheless, her pain never subsided and progressed to 4/10 while sitting and 6/10 with walking for longer than 1 h. The patient did not experience pain with initiation of gait nor was there appreciable nighttime discomfort.

On physical examination, the patient stood 5 feet and 3 inches tall weighing 110 pounds and walked with a non-antalgic, even gait. Trendelenburg, straight leg raise, and Stinchfield tests were negative bilaterally. Range of motion of both hips was symmetric with 120° flexion, 70° external rotation, 45° internal rotation, 60° abduction, and 20° adduction. There was a positive anterior impingement test as pain was elicited at the extremes of flexion and internal rotation of the right hip. She was neurovascularly intact.

Diagnosis/Assessment

AP and oblique radiographs of the right hip demonstrated prior decompression tracts and sclerosis of the femoral head consistent with ON (Fig. 10.1a, b). These radiographs further showed adequate joint space and a grossly spherical femoral head. The decision was made to obtain higher resolution imaging; however, the patient's severe kidney disease precluded the use of IV contrast. Therefore, the hip was further evaluated with a 3 Tesla MRI, which was also able to detect a 1 cm^2 focal area of femoral head collapse within the weight-bearing zone and loss of overlying articular cartilage (Fig. 10.2a, b). The shape of the image was of particular interest and was located superior to the previously made core tract. The remainder of the imaging assessment was unremarkable; in particular, she did not have evidence of labral pathology.

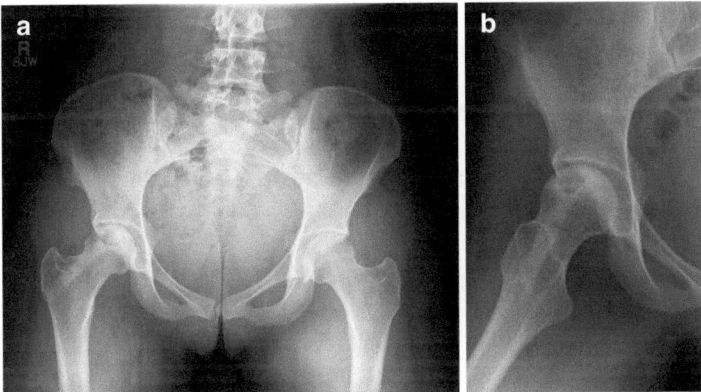

FIGURE 10.1 Preoperative AP (**a**) and oblique (**b**) radiographs of the right hip showing a previous core decompression tract with sclerotic changes consistent with ON. The femoral head appears spherical

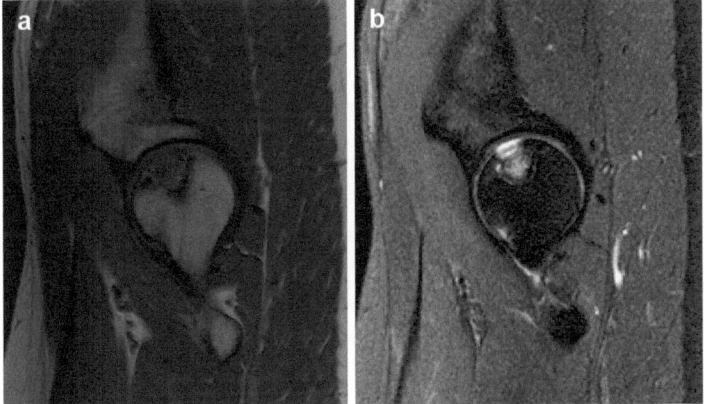

FIGURE 10.2 Preoperative 3 Tesla MRI images (**a, b**) showing a focal 1 cm^2 collapsed osteonecrotic lesion in the superior weight-bearing zone of the femoral head with overlying loss of articular cartilage

Given the patient's progressive pain, physical examination, and imaging findings, the decision was made to pursue operative intervention. Total hip arthroplasty provides the most predictable option for pain relief in the setting of ON with femoral head collapse. However, this patient's young age, well-controlled nephropathy without continued use of steroids, and small, focal area of femoral head damage presented a unique opportunity for further joint preservation. After being presented with both options and the inherent risks and benefits unique to each procedure, she elected to undergo surgical dislocation, assessment of the lesion, and potential OATS.

Management

Through a straight skin incision laterally, the fascia was split to access the posterior aspect of the greater trochanter. A trochanteric flip osteotomy was performed with a subsequent distal subvastus approach to the femur. The greater trochanteric piece was flipped anteriorly, and care was taken to break the anterior aspect of the fragment for later repositioning. The interval between the piriformis and gluteus minimus was dissected, and a complete capsule exposure was performed in a Z-shaped fashion to gain access anteriorly, superiorly, and posteriorly. Care was taken not to injure the labrum proximally and at the level of the rim. On the femoral side, she had a well-circumscribed defect measuring 1 cm^2 (Fig. 10.3a). Inferior and medially on the femoral head, there was an extension of the cartilage around Weitbrecht's ligament that would serve as a donor site. Using the OATS instrumentation, a 1 × 1 cm cartilage and bony plug was extracted. A 1 cm OATS cylinder extractor was used to create a similar defect at the level of the recipient site with a depth of 1 cm (Fig. 10.3b). This process exposed fresh bleeding bone; additional burring at the recipient site was carried out to debride dead surrounding bone. The 1 × 1 cm osteochondral graft was then placed into the defect, which achieved acceptable press-fit fixation (Fig. 10.3c). Cylinders of bone were then taken from the trochanteric bed and used to fill the inferior medial donor site. The hip was reduced and carried through a range of motion, which was quite smooth. The trochanteric flip osteotomy was reduced and fixed with three screws.

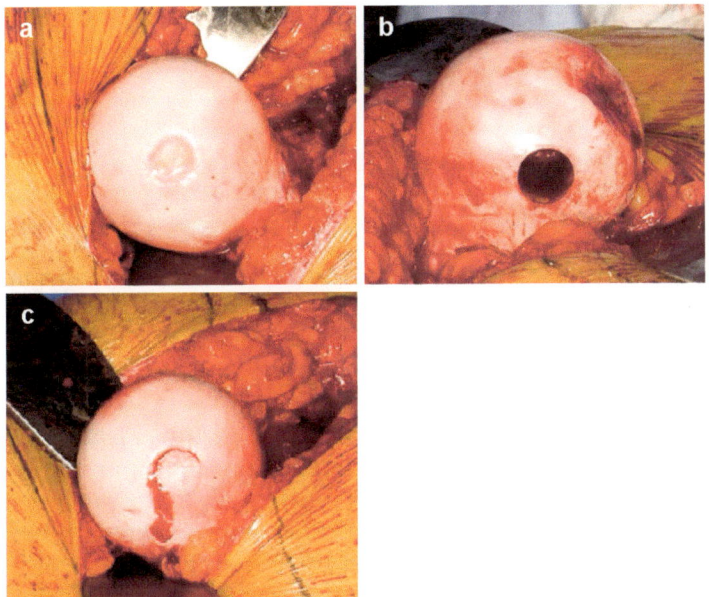

FIGURE 10.3 Intraoperative photographs showing the focal osteone-crotic lesion on the femoral head (**a**), resection of the lesion using the OATS cylinder extractor (**b**), and press-fit placement of an osteochondral autograft cylinder derived from the inferior medial femoral head using the OATS technology (**c**)

In summary, this patient received:

1. Surgical dislocation of the right hip
2. Resection of a 1 cm^2 cylinder of necrotic bone and degen-erated articular cartilage in the weight-bearing zone of the femoral head
3. Replacement of the resected area with a similarly sized osteochondral cylinder donated from the inferior medial femoral head using OATS instrumentation
4. Replacement of the donor site on the femoral head with a similarly sized core of bone from the greater trochanteric bed
5. Fixation of the trochanteric flip osteotomy with triple screw fixation

She was managed postoperatively with toe touch weight bearing for 8 weeks and advancement to full weight bearing thereafter.

Outcome

This 25-year-old woman with a failed core decompression for corticosteroid-induced ON of the femoral head was treated successfully with surgical dislocation and OATS for a 1 cm^2 area that was believed to be head penetration from a previous decompression. Her trochanteric hardware was removed at 2 months postoperatively. At 1-year follow-up, her groin pain remained absent, and radiographs demonstrated a spherical femoral head with partial resolution of cystic changes (Fig. 10.4a, b). She continues abductor strengthening and stretching for mild peri-trochanteric pain and will be seen at routine follow-up time points.

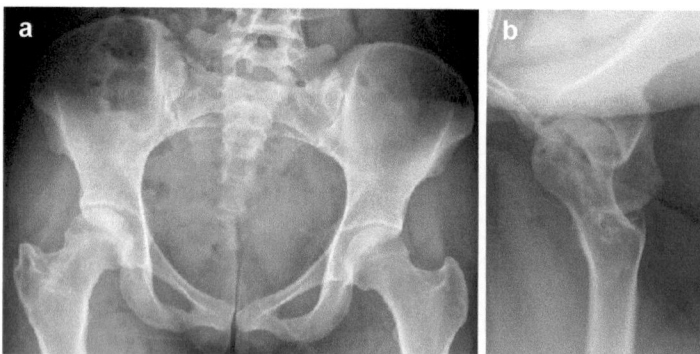

FIGURE 10.4 One-year postoperative AP (**a**) and lateral (**b**) radiographs of the right hip showing changes consistent with previous trochanteric osteotomy and hardware. The ON has not progressed and some previous cystic changes have resolved. Femoral head integrity is maintained

Literature Review

Currently the literature is restricted to small and heterogeneous case reports of osteochondral autograft transplantation for the management of ON of the femoral head. The current literature is discussed in Chapter 14. Early reports indicate that this technique can be successfully applied as a temporizing measure for disease progression in carefully selected patients with small lesions. However, until longer term, more robust studies potentially show otherwise, these procedures should be regarded as temporary joint preservation strategies to delay total hip replacement in young and active patients.

The purpose of the current chapter was to demonstrate the treatment of what was a potential complication associated with core decompression. In light of the lesion size and perfect symmetrical shape, the most plausible explanation for its occurrence was penetration of the femoral head with the decompression device. This can be avoided with careful advancement of the drill over a guidewire if necessary and verification on biplanar fluoroscopy. It is often seen that the drill comes in closer proximity to the articular surface on the frog leg lateral than on the AP fluoroscopic imaging, and therefore advancement of the drill on the lateral position may potentially avoid penetration.

In regard to the treatment with OATS, one previous study followed 20 patients (21 hips) that used two treatment protocols: (1) OATS for small precollapse ARCO stage IIA or IIB lesions or (2) OATS augmented with morselized bone allograft for large precollapse ARCO stage IIC or postcollapse ARCO stage III and IV lesions [1]. The group treated with OATS alone included seven hips followed for a mean of 46 months; one patient (14%) progressed to require total hip replacement. The group treated with OATS augmented with morselized bone allograft included 13 hips followed for a mean of 33 months; five patients (38%) progressed to require total hip replacement. This report has many limitations, but seems to intuitively indicate that OATS is more successfully applied in small ON lesions of the femoral head and the lesion in this case was both small in size and had underlying osteonecrosis.

Clinical Pearls and Pitfalls

- In this case, an OATS procedure was used to salvage a complication occurring from treatment of osteone-crosis of the femoral head.
- The necrotic area below must be resected until cir-cumferential bleeding bone is exposed to potentiate autograft ingrowth and stability.
- Autograft bone from the trochanter can be used to elevate the depth of the lesion if the plug requires support from within the head.
- The donor osteochondral graft must match the size of the resected lesion as closely as possible with the goal of achieving press-fit transplantation. The cir-cumference of the lesion also needs to match as close as possible to the circumference of the recipient site.

References

1. Gagala J, Tarczynska M, Gaweda K. Clinical and radiological out-comes of treatment of avascular necrosis of the femoral head using autologous osteochondral transfer (mosaicplasty): prelimi-nary report. International orthopaedics. 2013;37(7):1239–44.

Part II
Late Pre-Collapse or
Post-Collapse: Head Preserving

Chapter 11
Nonvascularized Bone Grafting

Todd P. Pierce, Julio J. Jauregui, Jeffrey J. Cherian,
Randa K. Elmallah, and Michael A. Mont

Case Presentation

A 23-year-old man who had a history of sickle cell disease presented with a history of left hip pain. His pain crisis events typically occur around his shoulders and hips. He has no other past medical history.

Diagnosis/Assessment

Radiographs confirmed left hip Ficat stage III. On examination, he had normal muscle tone and strength (see Fig. 11.1).

T.P. Pierce, MD • J.J. Jauregui, MD • J.J. Cherian, DO
R.K. Elmallah, MD • M.A. Mont, MD (✉)
Center for Joint Preservation and Replacement, Rubin Institute
for Advanced Orthopaedics, Sinai Hospital of Baltimore,
2401 West Belvedere Avenue, Baltimore, MD, USA
e-mail: tpierce@gwmail.gwu.edu; juljau@gmail.com;
jjaicherian@gmail.com; randaelmallah@gmail.com;
mmont@lifebridgehealth.org; rhondamont@aol.com

R.J. Sierra (ed.), *Osteonecrosis of the Femoral Head*,   117
DOI 10.1007/978-3-319-50664-7_11,
© Mayo Foundation for Medical Education and Research 2017

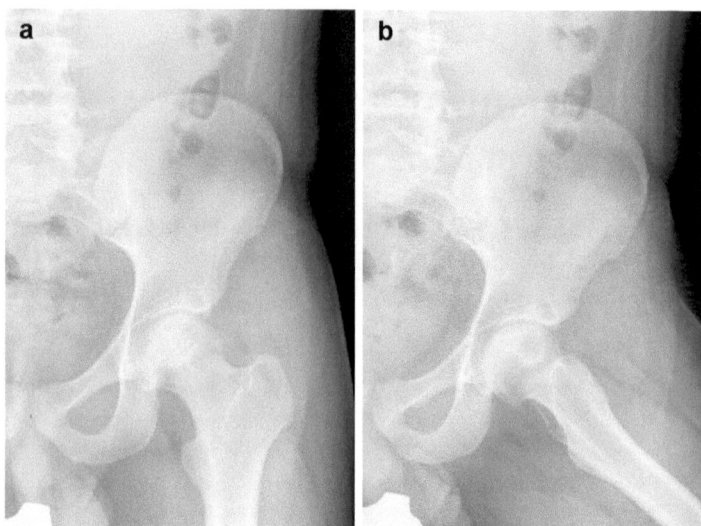

FIGURE 11.1 (**a, b**) Preoperative radiographs showing Ficat stage II sclerotic osteonecrotic lesions with no signs of femoral head collapse

Management

After consultation with the patient regarding the risks, benefits, and alternatives of various treatment options, it was decided that he would undergo left hip nonvascularized bone grafting with cancellous bone chips. Informed consent was obtained after discussing the risks and benefits of the planned procedures prior to surgery.

Bone Graft

After adequate spinal anesthesia, we prepared and draped the left hip in the usual aseptic manner. A 12 cm incision was made using the anterior-lateral approach, was continued into, and incised through the fascia lata. The anterior 40% of the gluteus medius and minimus was detached, a capsulectomy was performed, and the femoral neck was exposed. There was 1 mm collapse of the femoral head. Using an osteotome, we then made a 2 × 2 cm femoral neck window anteriorly. Using an 8 mm burr, we drilled out the necrotic bone until we observed viable bleeding bone. After elevation of the cartilage, the femoral head defect was packed with a combination of bone morphogenic proteins (BMPs) and corticocancellous (allograft) bone chips from the hospital blood bank. The window was then fixed using three pins, and the wound was irrigated carefully to ensure that no BMP remained within the soft tissue. After closure of the muscles, subcutaneous tissue, and skin, a dressing was applied. The patient was brought back to the recovery room in a stable condition. He was discharged with instructions to bear 25% of weight on the left lower extremity. At 6 weeks, he was allowed 50% weight bearing until 10 weeks when he was advanced to full weight bearing.

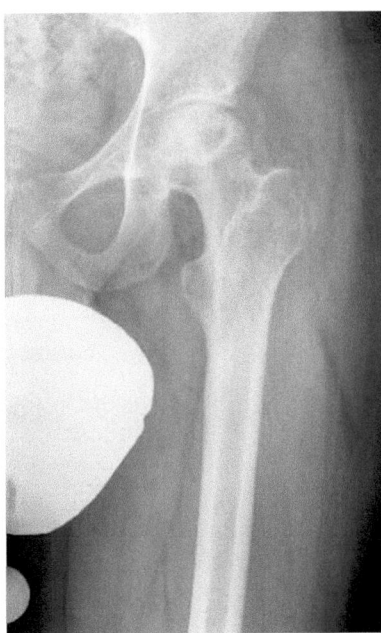

FIGURE 11.2 7-year post-bone grafting showing stable osteo-necrotic lesions without signs of disease progression

Outcome

The patient was followed up for 7 years annually, and radiographs obtained at last follow-up showed no evidence of any collapse, fracture, or dislocation (see Fig. 11.2). He had no complaints, minimal discomfort, and full range of motion in his hip, and he was able to successfully perform all activities of daily living.

Clinical Pearls and Pitfalls

- Consideration must be given to the technique used when trying to avoid complications:
  - Lightbulb procedure
    - Use an osteotome to perfect the cortical window.
    - If the femoral head is penetrated with the burr or curette, the patient should be converted to a THA.
  - Trapdoor procedure
    - Dislocate the femoral head and create a window through the collapsed articular cartilage.
    - Create a flap from the chondral surface, allowing for necrotic bone removal.
    - If no bleeding bone is present, the patient should be converted to a THA.
- We prefer capsulectomy over capsulotomy, as we have seen that those who have had a capsulotomy occasionally present with symptoms secondary to the development of scar tissue.
- There should always be the appropriate equipment to convert to a THA if necessary.

- Avoid penetrating the acetabular labrum during the anterior capsulectomy as this may result in pain and instability.
- The hip abductors must be repaired meticulously when concluding the procedure to minimize the risk of instability. If the repair is not adequate, the patient may exhibit a Trendelenburg gait.

Bibliography

1. Zhang HJ, Liu YW, Du ZQ, Guo H, Fan KJ, Liang GH, Liu XC. Therapeutic effect of minimally invasive decompression combined with impaction bone grafting on osteonecrosis of the femoral head. Eur J Orthop Surg Traumatol. 2013;23(8):913.
2. Gagala J, Tarczynska M, Gaweda K, Matuszewski L. The use of osteochondral allograft with bone marrow-derived mesenchymal cells and hinge joint distraction in the treatment of post-collapse stage of osteonecrosis of the femoral head. Med Hypotheses. 2014;83(3):398.
3. Wang BL, Sun W, Shi ZC, Zhang NF, Yue DB, Guo WS, Shi SH, Li ZR. Treatment of nontraumatic osteonecrosis of the femoral head using bone impaction grafting through a femoral neck window. Int Orthop. 2010;34(5):635.
4. Seyler TM, Marker DR, Ulrich SD, Fatscher T, Mont MA. Nonvascularized bone grafting defers joint arthroplasty in hip osteonecrosis. Clin Orthop Relat Res. 2008;466(5):1125.
5. Mont MA, Etienne G, Ragland PS. Outcome of nonvascularized bone grafting for osteonecrosis of the femoral head. Clin Orthop Relat Res. 2003;417(417):84.
6. Mont MA, Einhorn TA, Sponseller PD, Hungerford DS. The trapdoor procedure using autogenous cortical and cancellous bone grafts for osteonecrosis of the femoral head. J Bone Joint Surg Br. 1998;80(1):56.

Chapter 12
Bilateral Nonvascularized Bone Grafting

Todd P. Pierce, Julio J. Jauregui, Jeffrey J. Cherian, Randa K. Elmallah, and Michael A. Mont

Case Presentation

A 39-year-old man with history of an unknown autoimmune disorder presented to the office with bilateral hip pain. It is most pronounced with any physical activity, particularly with ascending stairs. He has been under the care of a rheumatologist and a primary care physician for this pain, and conservative treatment modalities have resulted in minimal relief.

T.P. Pierce, MD • J.J. Jauregui, MD • J.J. Cherian, DO
R.K. Elmallah, MD • M.A. Mont, MD (✉)
Center for Joint Preservation and Replacement, Rubin Institute for Advanced Orthopaedics, Sinai Hospital of Baltimore, 2401 West Belvedere Avenue, Baltimore, MD 21215, USA
e-mail: tpierce@gwmail.gwu.edu; juljau@gmail.com; jjaicherian@gmail.com; randaelmallah@gmail.com; mmont@lifebridgehealth.org; rhondamont@aol.com

R.J. Sierra (ed.), *Osteonecrosis of the Femoral Head*,
DOI 10.1007/978-3-319-50664-7_12,
© Mayo Foundation for Medical Education and Research 2017

Diagnosis/Assessment

Radiographs confirmed bilateral stage III osteonecrosis with Kerboul medium-sized lesion with 2 mm of collapse on the left. On the right, there was a Kerboul small-sized lesion with approximately 1 mm of head collapse. On examination, he had normal muscle tone and strength. Given his clinical exam, his young age, and the fact his collapse did not extended beyond 2 mm, the decision was made proceed with bilateral hip bone grafting. Our plan was to complete bone grafting on the right first and proceed with the left approximately 2 weeks following.

Management

Right Hip Bone Grafting

The patient was brought into the operating room and, after adequate anesthesia, placed in the left lateral decubitus position. We prepared and draped the right hip in the usual aseptic manner. We used the anterolateral approach, made a 12 cm incision, and dissected through skin and subcutaneous tissue. We then deepened the incision through the fascia lata and detached the anterior 40% of the gluteus medius and minimus. We then completed a capsulectomy.

During this time, the patient had a marked amount of the bleeding, but we were able to achieve hemostatic control with electrocautery. Because of this bleeding, we felt that it was more appropriate to do one side and proceed with bone grafting on the contralateral side after 2 weeks. The hip was then exposed without dislocating it. An approximately 2 × 2 cm window at the femoral head and neck junction was made using an oscillating saw. We burred out the femoral head under fluoroscopic control. We were able to see that we got a good removal of the dead bone.

We then packed this window with a combination of the patient's bone marrow from the iliac crest, BMPs, and allograft bone, and we layered that in place. The window was then fixed with three pins. After careful irrigation, closure of the muscles, subcutaneous tissue, and skin was performed. A sterile dressing was applied, and the patient was brought back to the recovery room in stable condition.

Two weeks later, we proceeded with the left hip bone grafting treating it in the same fashion as the right.

Outcome

Approximately 10 years after his bone grafting procedures, the patient was doing well. He was ambulating without any assistive devices at this time and did not require any pain medications. Radiographic evaluation showed no progression of disease, and the known osteonecrotic lesions were stable (see Fig. 12.1). On physical exam, he had good range of motion and was neurovascularly intact bilaterally.

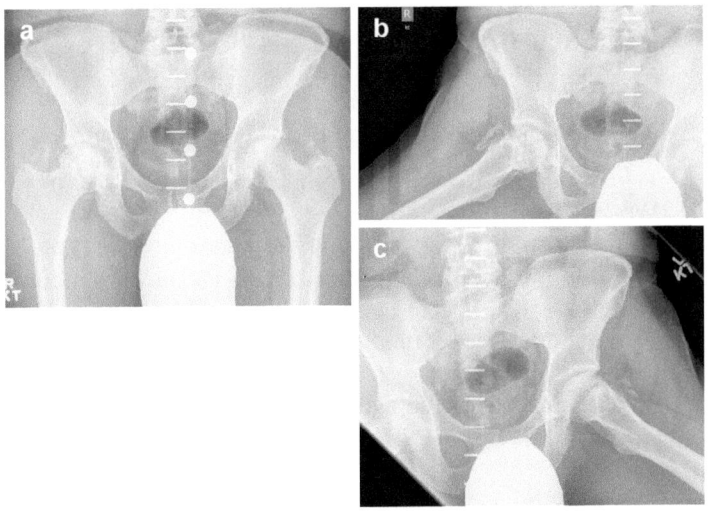

FIGURE 12.1 (**a–c**) Radiographs of post-bilateral grafting showing Ficat stage III disease of the right hip and stage II disease in the left hip without signs of progression of the lesions from preoperative radiographs

Literature Review

There are multiple small studies displaying the efficacy of nonvascularized bone grafting in conjunction with core decompression (see Table 12.1). In general, most of the studies support the use of this technique in pre-collapse stages of ON.

Clinical Pearls and Pitfalls

- Consideration must be given to the technique used when trying to avoid complications.
  - Lightbulb procedure
    - Use an osteotome to perfect the cortical window.
    - If the femoral head is penetrated with the burr or curette, the patient should be converted to a THA.
  - Trapdoor procedure
    - Dislocate the femoral head and create a window through the collapsed articular cartilage.
    - Create a flap from the chondral surface, allowing for necrotic bone removal.
    - If no bleeding bone is present, the patient should be converted to a THA.
- We prefer capsulectomy over capsulotomy, as we have seen that those who have had a capsulotomy occasionally present with symptoms secondary to the development of scar tissue.
- There should always be the appropriate equipment to convert to a THA if necessary.
- Avoid penetrating the acetabular labrum during the anterior capsulectomy as this may result in pain and instability.
- The hip abductors must be repaired meticulously when concluding the procedure to minimize the risk of instability. If the repair is not adequate, the patient may exhibit a Trendelenburg gait.

TABLE 12.1 Outcomes of nonvascularized bone grafting

Author, year	Number of hips	Surgical technique	Bone graft	Stages	Mean follow-up, months (range)	Mean postoperative HHS, points	Conversion to THA; %
Zhang et al. [1], (2013)	85	Lightbulb	Autograft ilium	ARCO IC–IIIC	– (24 to –)	86.4	7
Gagala et al. [2], (2013)	13	Trapdoor	Allograft lateral femoral condyle	ARCO II–IV	33 (18–75)	87.9	38
Wang et al. [3], (2010)	138	Lightbulb	Autograft ilium (cortico-cancellous)	ARCO IIA–IIIA	25.4 (7–42)	79	–
Seyler et al. [4], (2008)	39	Trapdoor	Cancellous bone chips; BMP-7	Ficat II–III	36 (24–50)	75	33
Mont et al. [5], (2003)	21	Lightbulb	Allograft bone	Steinberg II–IV	48 (36–55)	91	14.3
Mont et al. [6], (1998)	30	Trapdoor	Autograft ilium (cortico-cancellous)	Ficat stage III and IV	56 (30–60)	92	6.7

IT intertrochanteric

References

1. Zhang HJ, Liu YW, Du ZQ, Guo H, Fan KJ, Liang GH, Liu XC. Therapeutic effect of minimally invasive decompression combined with impaction bone grafting on osteonecrosis of the femoral head. Eur J Orthop Surg Traumatol. 2013;23(8):913.
2. Gagala J, Tarczynska M, Gaweda K, Matuszewski L. The use of osteochondral allograft with bone marrow-derived mesenchymal cells and hinge joint distraction in the treatment of post-collapse stage of osteonecrosis of the femoral head. Med Hypotheses. 2014;83(3):398.
3. Wang BL, Sun W, Shi ZC, Zhang NF, Yue DB, Guo WS, Shi SH, Li ZR. Treatment of nontraumatic osteonecrosis of the femoral head using bone impaction grafting through a femoral neck window. Int Orthop. 2010;34(5):635.
4. Seyler TM, Marker DR, Ulrich SD, Fatscher T, Mont MA. Nonvascularized bone grafting defers joint arthroplasty in hip osteonecrosis. Clin Orthop Relat Res. 2008;466(5):1125.
5. Mont MA, Etienne G, Ragland PS. Outcome of nonvascularized bone grafting for osteonecrosis of the femoral head. Clin Orthop Relat Res. 2003;417(417):84.
6. Mont MA, Einhorn TA, Sponseller PD, Hungerford DS. The trap-door procedure using autogenous cortical and cancellous bone grafts for osteonecrosis of the femoral head. J Bone Joint Surg Br. 1998;80(1):56.

Chapter 13
Femoral Head Decompression Using the X-REAM® Followed by Autologous Tibial Cancellous Bone Impaction

Stefan B. Keizer and Rob G.H.H. Nelissen

Case Presentation

A 50-year-old woman presented to the orthopaedic outpatient department with 2½ year history of progressive hip pain on the left side. She had a history of a hemithyroidectomy, a cataract operation and meningitis 8 years before, for which she had received high-dose steroids during a short period of time. Two years before

S.B. Keizer, MD (✉)
Department of Orthopaedics, Haaglanden Medical Center,
The Hague, The Netherlands
e-mail: s.keizer@mchaaglanden.nl

R.G.H.H. Nelissen, MD, PhD
Department of Orthopaedics, Leiden University Medical Center,
Leiden, The Netherlands

R.J. Sierra (ed.), *Osteonecrosis of the Femoral Head*,
DOI 10.1007/978-3-319-50664-7_13,
© Mayo Foundation for Medical Education and Research 2017

her consultation, osteonecrosis of the hip was diagnosed in another hospital treated with NSAIDs, resulting in pain relief for some time. Since she had progressive pain, she was referred to our institution. At her consultation she used a cane, was able to walk for only 10 min and used daily NSAIDs but no other medication. There was no history of alcohol or drug abuse.

Diagnosis/Assessment

On physical examination we saw a healthy 50-year-old woman with a BMI of 23. As for the hip, no Trendelenburg sign was present. She had painful and limited range of motion with a flexion of 90°, full extension, an external rotation of 20° and an internal rotation of 10°. Neurovascular assessment was normal. A frog leg and AP pelvis radiograph revealed a spherical femoral head with mottled osteoporotic and sclerotic areas involving the anterolateral aspect of the femoral head. There was no crescent sign (Fig. 13.1).

A MRI showed the anterolateral lesion in the femoral head, consistent with an osteonecrosis of the hip, Steinberg stage IIB (Fig. 13.2).

Management

In our institution we use the Steinberg classification to make a choice between the different treatment options. In this classification we mainly use the pre- and post-collapse stages to differentiate between the treatment options. In patients with a crescent sign at the femoral head, the size of the lesion, age of the patient and the continuous use of steroids are taken in account. In general, the necrotic bone decompression and removal, succeeded by the autologous impaction grafting technique, is used for stages 1 and 2. In young patients (<40 years), we consider the decompression and impaction

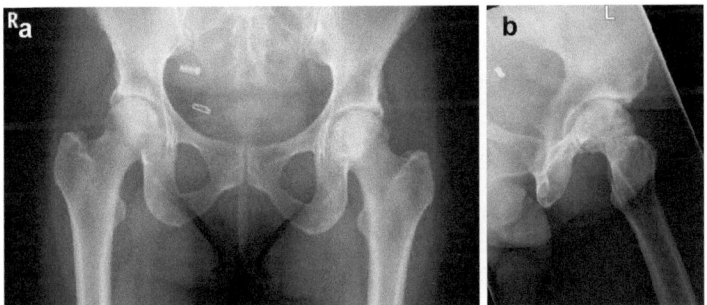

FIGURE 13.1 (**a**) AP view of the pelvis: radiolucencies of both femoral heads with curvilinear sclerosis. (**b**) Lateral view shows spherical contours of the femoral heads

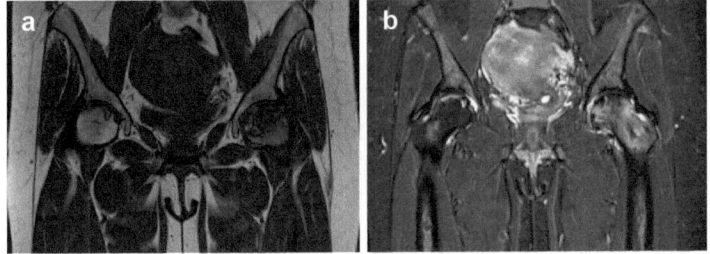

FIGURE 13.2 (**a**) On T1-weighted coronal MR image, circumscribed "band-like" lesions with low signal intensity are noted in both femoral heads. (**b**) Joint and diffuse bone marrow oedema of the left femoral head and neck are demonstrated on T2-weighted fat-suppressed coronal MR image

technique also in stage 3 when there is a small area of femoral head osteonecrosis (stage 3a). As of stage 3a and higher, we advise a THA.

Background

Our treatment of ONFH with decompression and autologous bone impaction grafting is an evolution of our prior treatments using decompression and structural cortical bone grafts and autologous cancellous bone grafts of the femoral head. In the 1980s we started treating ONFH with the Phemister technique [1]. This technique removes the necrotic subchondral bone, and then grafting of the lesion is performed with autologous cancellous bone of the proximal tibia and the placement of an autologous cortical tibia graft in the femoral neck and head. Because of the donor side morbidity of the cortical graft (i.e. tibial fractures) seen with this procedure, we started using a fibular allograft and cancellous bone from the greater trochanter region.

The results of these techniques showed that the results were better with autologous cortical tibia graft versus the fibular allograft technique [2].

The difference in survival between the two grafting techniques (autologous cortical versus allograft cortical), despite the use of cancellous autograft in both techniques, was thought to be of the results of the autologous cancellous bone of the proximal tibia, which was reasoned to have better osteoinductive qualities compared to the trochanteric region, which is supported by others [3].

The position of a strut of a fibula or tibia had a minimal effect on the outcome of the procedure, since there was no correlation between the position of the graft in the subchondral femoral head and the revision rate [2].

Evaluation of these study results was pivotal for developing our current treatment policy and surgical technique, in which we decompress and remove the necrotic bone with a special percutaneous expandable reamer the X-REAM® (Wright Medical Technology, Inc., Arlington, TN). After which we impact the lesion with autologous cancellous bone obtained from the proximal tibia.

Description of Surgical Procedure

The patient is placed in the supine position on the fracture (i.e. surgical table with independent movable table blades for the legs, which are also radiolucent). First, cancellous bone graft is collected from the proximal tibia. An inverted L-shaped incision is made utilizing a lateral approach to the proximal tibia. The transverse limb of the incision is 2 cm distal to the lateral joint line. The vertical limb is midline to the tibia and carried 8 cm distally. The incision is carried down to periosteum with the lateral portion of the tibia expose by lifting off the anterior tibial muscle from the lateral cortex of the tibia. A cortical window is made of 1 medial to lateral by 5 cm proximal to distal and cancellous bone is harvested from the proximal tibia with a 5 to 8 mm curette. Care is taken that bone removal stops at least 2 cm from the joint line of the tibial plateau to prevent fractures. After the removal of the cancellous bone, the cortical window is replaced and the fascia of the anterior tibial muscle is closed.

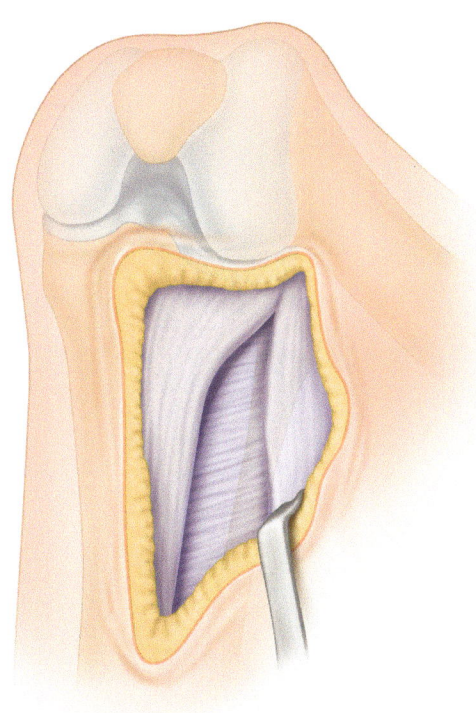

Secondly a 5 cm long lateral skin incision is made just distal to the greater trochanter. The fascia lata is split in the direction of the skin incision, and the vastus lateralis muscle is lifted off from the lateral cortex of the femur following L-shaped incision of the muscle. Under fluoroscopy a guide pin is inserted towards the centre of osteonecrosis (usually anterolateral) until it is seated in the subchondral bone area. The preoperative MRI images are also used for the most optimal position of this guide pin. Using a 9 mm cannulated drill bit, an intraosseous tunnel reaching the osteonecrotic area is created. Advanced debridement of the osteonecrotic area is carried out using the X-REAM® percutaneous expandable reamer. Care is taken not to violate the subchondral plate with the blades of the reamer.

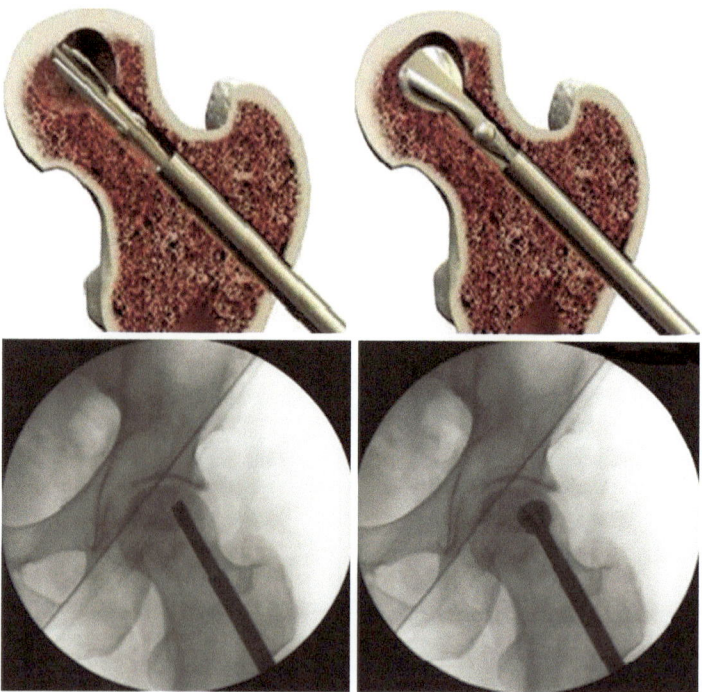

After all necrotic bone is removed with the X-REAM®, the lesion and tunnel is washed out with pulse lavage of saline fluid. The autologous cancellous bone from the proximal tibia is then impacted layer by layer into the defect of femoral head. The remaining tunnel in the femoral neck is impacted with fresh-frozen cancellous allograft bone. Lastly, soft tissues including the vastus lateralis and fascia lata are repaired layer by layer.

Postoperative Rehabilitation Plan

During the first 6 weeks after surgery, 15% weight bearing on the operated leg with two crutches is allowed. After that period patients progressed to full weight bearing as tolerated in 6-week time. The main purpose of the postoperative physical therapy is to regain the stability whilst walking and explain closed chain muscle strengthening exercises. There is no limitation of the range of motion of the hip, and at 6 weeks postoperatively, the patient is allowed to return to their normal activities and work. In our opinion, patients are able to decide when to increase activities using pain as guidance as to progressive weight bearing during activities.

Outcome

At 3 months after surgery, the preoperative pain level of this 50-year-old patient with a Steinberg IIb osteonecrosis of her left femoral head has resolved. She was walking without any aid and at that time she was no longer on regular painkillers (Fig. 13.3).

One year after surgery, she had occasionally groin pain but could walk an unlimited distance without any support. The MRI showed a stable situation with no more bone marrow oedema and presence of a spherical femoral head (Fig. 13.4).

At 5-year follow-up, she had a painless ROM and used paracetamol once a week after long walks but was able to walk and climb the stair unlimited with a HHS 85. Radiological result was excellent with no collapse of the femoral head, but she did have a little of arthritis that may account for some of her intermittent pain (Fig. 13.5).

Literature Review

The rationale of our treatment is twofold: (1) decompression of the necrotic femoral head by removal of necrotic bone in order to interrupt the cycle of ischemia and interosseous hypertension and (2) grafting the femoral head defect with

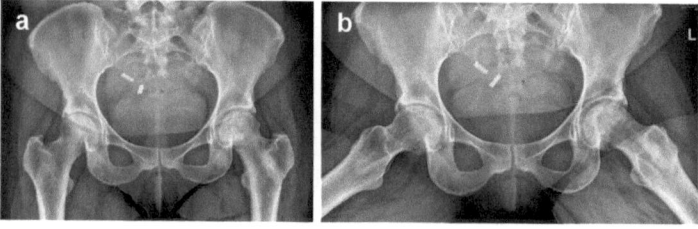

FIGURE 13.3 Three months postoperative. (**a**) AP view: visible core tract with impacted bone graft. (**b**) Frog leg view

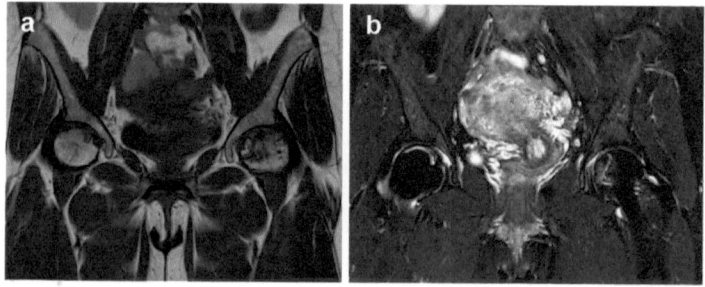

FIGURE 13.4 (**a**) On T1-weighted coronal MR image, smaller lesions with low signal intensity in the left femoral head. (**b**) No more bone marrow oedema of the left femoral head and neck on T2-weighted fat-suppressed coronal MR image

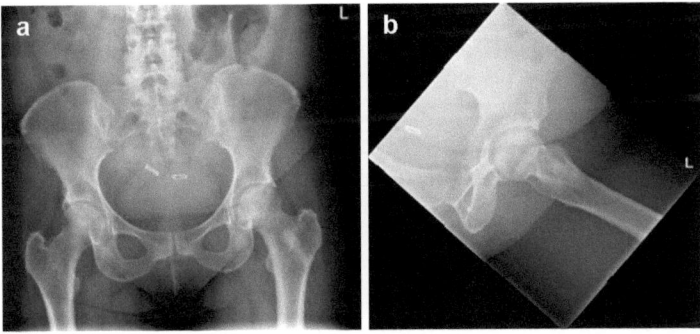

FIGURE 13.5 (**a**) AP view: no collapse or progression of the osteone-crosis of the femoral head. (**b**) Frog leg view: spherical femoral head

impacted autologous cancellous bone and the femoral neck with impacted allograft bone.

The effectiveness of these procedures may be related to pushing biology towards bone healing by removal of the large osteonecrotic area in the femoral head. Furthermore, the availability of autologous cytokines, BMPs and stem cells endowed with osteogenic properties present in the grafted bone will promote this osteogenesis of the former necrotic area [4, 5].

Hernigou et al. showed decreased activity of bone marrow cells in the intertrochanteric region and in the iliac crest in patients with osteonecrosis of the femoral head secondary to steroid therapy or alcohol abuse [3, 6].

In our not published series of 47 patients with ONFH of which 28 pre-collapse femoral heads (i.e. crescent sign, types II–III) were treated with the described technique of removal of necrotic bone and autologous bone impaction of the femo-ral head, the overall clinical (i.e. no collapse of femoral head) success rate was 75% at minimum 5-year follow-up. Patients with a collapse of the femoral head (Steinberg III) or larger osteonecrotic lesions had a higher rate of failure.

There are a few studies available on outcome after bone impaction grafting for the treatment of ONFH. Rijnen et al.

reported the first outcomes after bone impaction grafting in 28 hips with ONFH [7]. In that series, 14 hips (50%) had preoperative collapse of the femoral head. The overall clinical success rate was 64%, whereas 15 hips (54%) showed radiographic success at an average follow-up of 43 months. Patients older than 30 years, preoperative collapsed lesions and continued steroid use after surgery had a significantly higher likelihood of a radiographic and clinical failure.

Park et al. reported the outcome in 42 ONFH hips [8]. They showed an overall clinical and radiographic success rate of 74 and 50%, respectively. Worse outcome was associated with lesions >30% of the femoral head or a lateral location of the osteonecrotic area. In the study of Jung et al., these results were confirmed with report of 95 hips with ONFH. The overall clinical success rate was 78 and 46% radiographic success. They also concluded that a large or lateral lesion in the femoral head was associated with postoperative radiographic failure.

Clinical Pearls and Pitfalls

- The careful learning curve of this surgical technique alludes to the small balance between not over-impacting cancellous graft, causing subchondral bulging and even perforation of the subchondral plate, and also not under-impaction of the bone graft, which will lead to collapse of femoral head.
- As for the donor site morbidity, care should be taken to not remove bone less than 2 cm under the tibial plateau to prevent iatrogenic fractures. On average we impact 30 cc of bone graft into the head and an additional 20 to 30 cc into the core tract.
- Washing the cancellous graft appears to improve the mechanical properties, but because autograft contains osteoprogenitor cells and local growth factors to induce the mesenchymal cells to differentiate into mature osteoblasts, washing may remove beneficial

factors from the graft and lead to poorer incorporation. So we do not wash the autograft, but do wash the allograft bone.

- X-REAM® surgical instruments are very effective in removing a large volume of necrotic bone through a small cortical window.
- Some of the advantages of autologous bone grafting of the femoral head include stimulation and enhancing of bone repair following removal of the weak necrotic bone.
- Both the autologous and the allograft bone grafts are also scaffold for new bone to grow onto. Secondly the impacted bone grafts give structural stability of the excavated femoral head.
- Autologous cancellous bone of the proximal tibia is not only of better osteoinductive quality, but also a larger volume can be harvested from this area compared to the greater trochanteric region.

References

1. Phemister DB. Treatment of the necrotic head of the femur in adults. J Bone Joint Surg. 1949;31-A:55–66.
2. Keizer SB, Kock NB, Dijkstra PDS. Taminiau AHM Nelissen RGHH Treatment of osteonecrosis of the hip with a non-vascularized cortical graft. J Bone Joint Surg Br. 2006 Apr;88(4):460–6.
3. Hernigou P, Beaujean F. Abnormalities in the bone marrow of the iliac crest in patients who have osteonecrosis secondary to corticosteroid therapy or alcohol abuse. J Bone Joint Surg. 1997;79-A:1047–53.
4. Hauzeur JP, Pasteels JL. Pathology of bone marrow distant from the sequestrum in nontraumatic aseptic necrosis of the femoral head. In: Arlet J, Mazières B, editors. Bone circulation and bone necrosis. Berlin: Springer; 1990. p. 73–6.
5. Inoue A, Ono K. A histological study of idiopathic avascular necrosis of the head of the femur. J Bone Joint Surg. 1979;61-B:138–43.

6. Hernigou P, Beaujean F, Lambotte JC. Decrease in the mesenchymal stem-cell pool in the proximal femur in corticosteroid-induced osteonecrosis. J Bone Joint Surg Br. 1999;81:349–55.
7. Rijnen WH, Gardeniers JW, Buma P, Yamano K, Slooff TJ, Schreurs BW. Treatment of femoral head osteonecrosis using bone impaction grafting. Clin Orthop Relat Res. 2003;417:74–83.
8. Park YS, Rim YS, Park YK, Yun SH. Core decompression and impaction bone graft in avascular necrosis of the femoral head. J Korean Orthop Assoc. 1999;34:425–30.

Chapter 14
Autologous Osteochondral Transfer for Management of Femoral Head Osteonecrosis

J. Ryan Martin and Rafael J. Sierra

Case Presentation

S. M., a 25 y.o. female presented with several years of right hip pain. Two years prior to presenting to our institution, she underwent a right hip arthroscopy for impingement. Two months post-operatively she felt her hip sublux but did not have a true dislocation. Several months later, her hip pain increased and she was diagnosed with avascular necrosis of the femoral head (MRI images) (Ficat stage 2). She underwent a hip

J.R. Martin, MD (✉)
OrthoCarolina, Hip and Knee Surgeon, 710 Park Center Dr. #300,
Matthews, NC 28105, USA
e-mail: johrmart@gmail.com

R.J. Sierra, MD
Mayo Clinic, 200 1st St. SW, Rochester, MN 55905, USA

R.J. Sierra (ed.), *Osteonecrosis of the Femoral Head*,
DOI 10.1007/978-3-319-50664-7_14,
© Mayo Foundation for Medical Education and Research 2017

141

decompression using multiple 3.2 mm drill holes at the outside hospital. She noted a few months of decreased pain until she had an acute episode of pain and was diagnosed with collapse of the femoral head (Ficat stage 3).

She continued to have pain daily and had been severely limited from activities of daily living. She was an avid runner and was no longer able to run secondary to pain. She had taken NSAIDs, altered her activities, and had tried physical therapy with no relief in pain.

Diagnosis/Assessment

She was in no acute distress. She ambulated with an antalgic gait. Her neurovascular examination was within normal limits. She had three small well-healed incisions over her hip from a previous hip arthroscopy and a larger incision over her right greater trochanter. Hip range of motion was 0–100° with pain at extreme flexion. She had 40° of internal and external rotation. She had a positive Stinchfield examination. The rest of her examination was within normal limits.

Initial diagnostic MRI of the right hip shows right femoral head AVN with multiple areas of bony edema on the coronal and axial views. Note at this time there was no collapse of the femoral head.

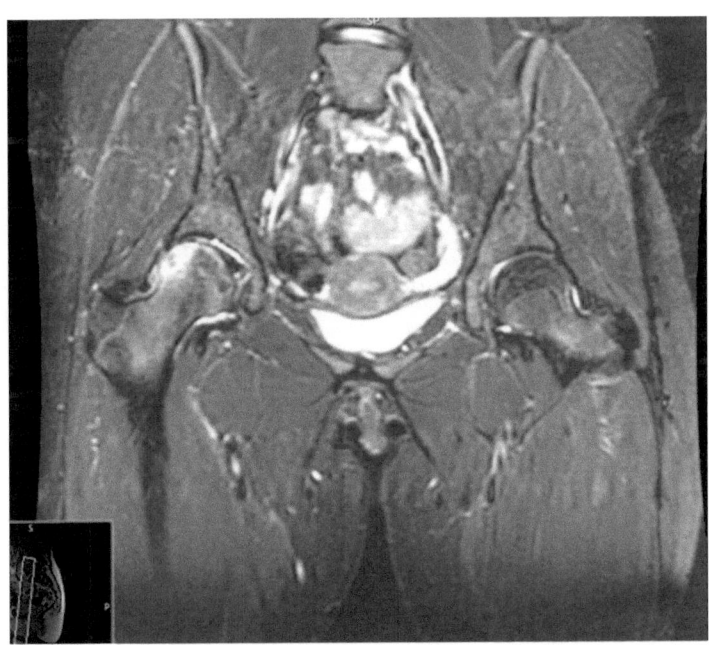

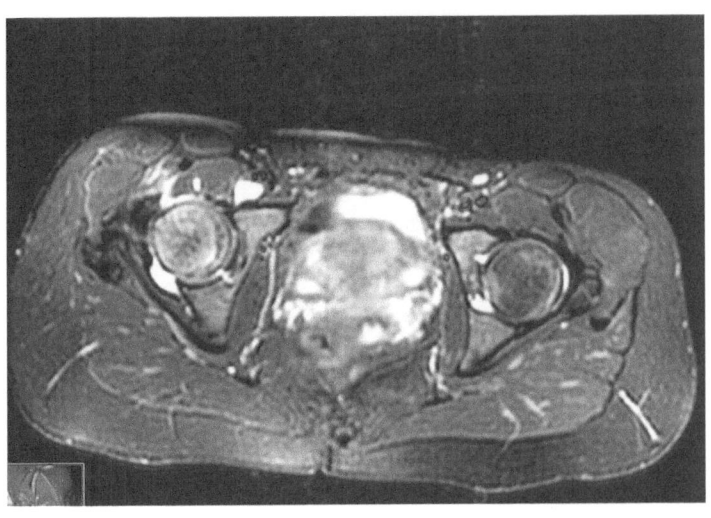

Preoperative X-rays: The AP and cross-table lateral radiograph of the right hip show a previous core decompression of the right hip with evidence of focal collapse of the superomedial femoral head

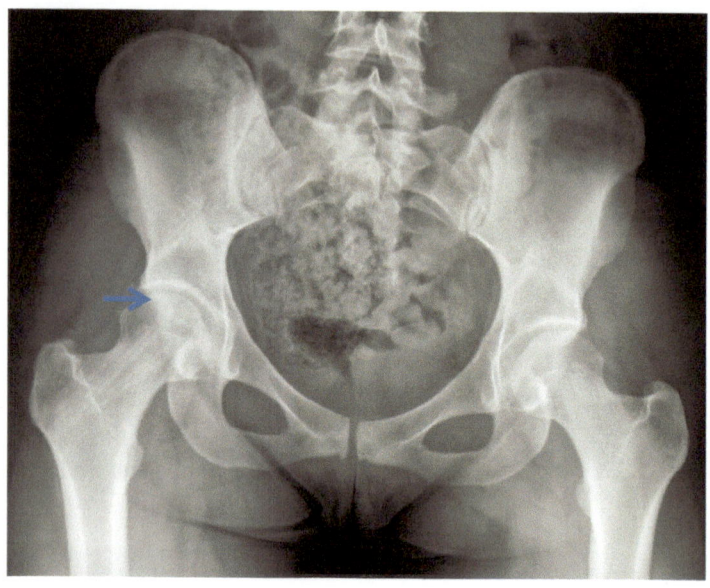

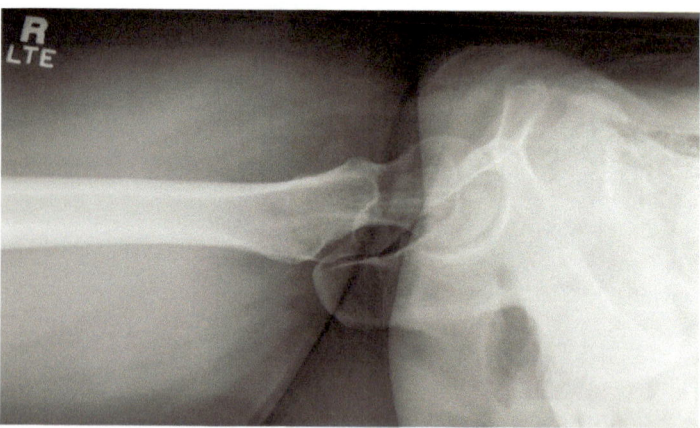

Management

A preoperative discussion was held with the patient to review the various treatment options. The two most commonly proposed options included nonoperative management vs. total hip arthroplasty. However, the patient had significant pain and wanted to return to running. For this reason, she did not feel that either option would allow her to return to her previous activity level. Because of the relatively small area of segmental collapse and relatively preserved acetabular cartilage, the decision was made to go ahead with joint preservation. The proposed procedure included a surgical hip dislocation; the approach would allow complete visualization of the femoral head and acetabulum and would give ample exposure to proceed with head-preserving procedures or THA if needed. We discussed osteochondral autograft transplantation of a non-weight-bearing portion of her femoral head to the area of AVN on her femoral head if the cartilage was found to be in poor condition vs. bone grafting and elevation of the necrotic segment if the cartilage was acceptable. A lateral skin incision was made centered over the greater trochanter on the patient's right hip. The fascia was split in line with the skin incision over the greater trochanter. A trochanteric flip osteotomy was performed from 5 mm anterior to the trochanteric overhang and directed distally and anteriorly exiting distal to the vastus ridge. A distal subvastus approach to the femur was carried out. The greater trochanteric piece was flipped anteriorly. Care was taken to break the anterior aspect of the fragment for later repositioning. The interval between the piriformis and gluteus minimus was dissected. A complete capsular exposure was performed. The entire anterior, superior, and posterior capsule was easily visualized utilizing this approach. A capsulotomy was carried out in a Z-shaped fashion. Care was taken not to injure the labrum proximally and at the level of the rim. Anterior and superior limbs of the capsule were then made. Distally we carried our capsulotomy to the level of the neck. The hip was dislocated with external rotation, and the foot was placed in an anterior position. She had damage to the anterosuperior acetabular cartilage. This entailed a delaminated area that measured approximately 1.5 cm × 4 mm in depth. The cartilage was of poor quality in this area. The acetabular cartilage damage was debrided and then the subchondral bone underwent microfracture. Attention was then turned to the femur. The patient had a large osteonecrotic lesion, which was adjacent to the fovea (Photos 1, 2, and 3). This measured at least 40 mm in diameter. The area of collapse was in the weight-bearing area of the femoral head. Three plugs of necrotic femoral head were removed from the area, each measuring 10 to 15 mm in depth (Photos 4 and 5). These three areas were then burred to a bleeding bony bed. Femoral bone cancellous autograft was harvested from the trochanteric bed where the trochanteric flip was performed and then placed into the depth of the osteochondral defect. Three osteochondral plugs were harvested from the lateral and anteromedial non-weight-bearing aspects of the femoral head. These measured, on average, between 6 and 11 mm in depth. These were then contoured to reconstruct the femoral head into the previous area of osteonecrosis. The osteochondral autograft appeared to sit flush in their receptor sites and were confirmed to have recontoured the head appropriately with an offset template (Photos 6 and 7). Bone marrow concentrate was injected under pressure into the femoral head through the fovea. Bone graft was then placed into the donor site, and it was felt that the femoral neck did not need screw fixation given the minimal bone graft taken. The hip was reduced and carried through a range of motion. The labrum appeared to be well reduced and stable to the rim where it was present. Intraoperative X-rays were obtained to evaluate the femoral head and placement of the trochanteric screws (intraoperative X-rays). Irrigation of the joint was carried out. The capsule was then closed with No. 1 Vicryl. The trochanteric flip osteotomy was reduced and fixed with three screws. The trochanteric bursa was closed over the screws. The fascia was closed with 0 Vicryl and 2-0 Monocryl in the subcutaneous tissue, and a 3-0 Monocryl was used to close the skin. The patient tolerated the procedure well and was transferred to the postoperative care unit in stable condition Figs. 14.1, 14.2, 14.3, 14.4, and 14.5.

Intraoperative X-rays: AP of the right hip with three screws into the greater trochanter for fixation of the osteotomy

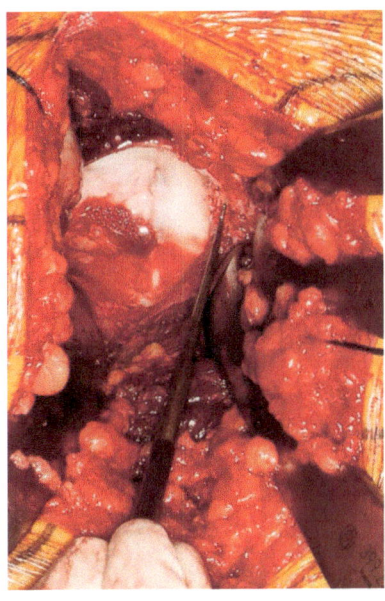

FIGURE 14.1 Intraoperative photograph zoomed in on the femoral head-neck junction. The labrum is being probed and noted to be in good condition

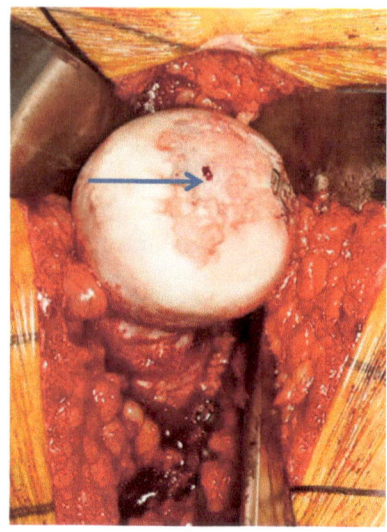

FIGURE 14.2 The femoral head has been dislocated and the osteonecrotic lesion is easily identified

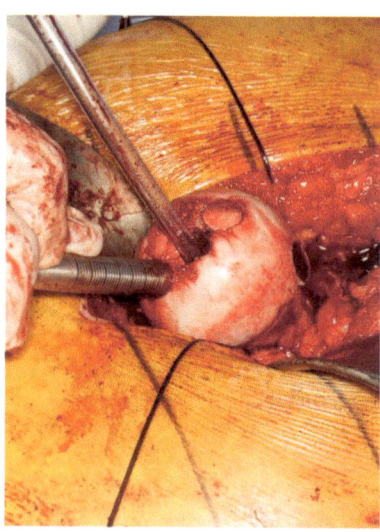

FIGURE 14.3 The osteonecrotic lesion is being prepared by removing the necrotic lesion and subsequently implanting normal osteochondral autograft from the non-weight-bearing donor site on the femoral head

FIGURE 14.4 Three donor osteochondral autografts have been taken from the non-weight-bearing aspect of the femoral head and transferred to the previous osteonecrotic region. We opted for only three plugs as we could not obtain other grafts from the donor site. The grafts were placed over the main weight-bearing area

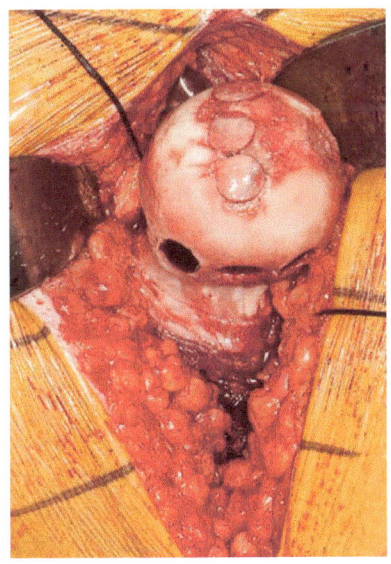

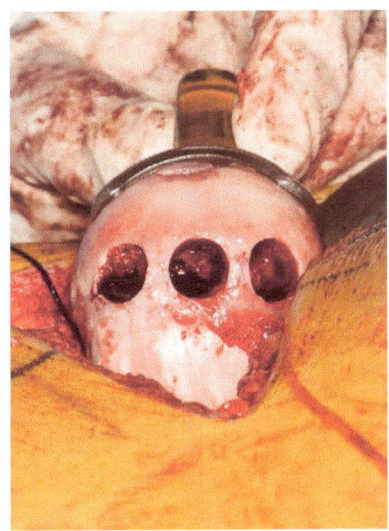

FIGURE 14.5 Concentricity of the femoral head is being assessed

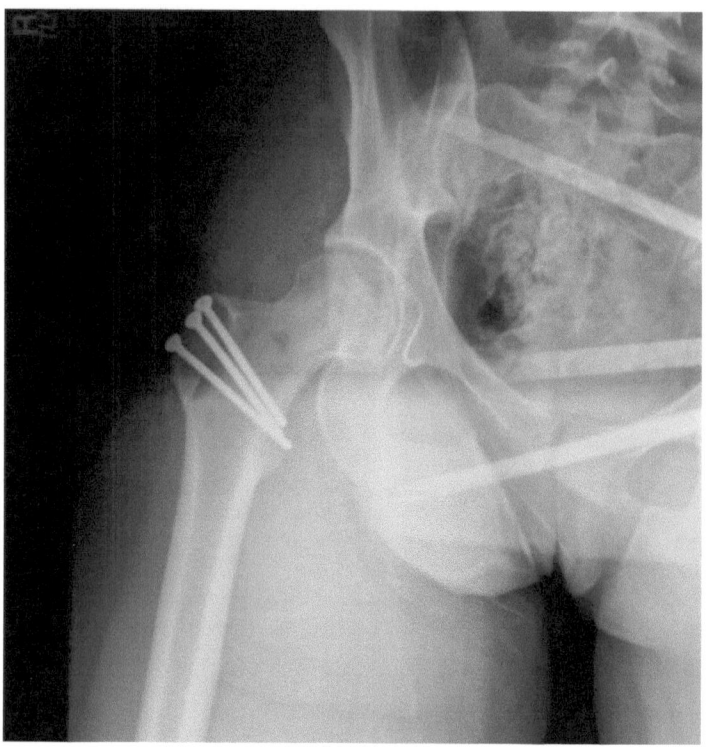

Outcome

She was admitted to the hospital for two nights and was discharged on oral pain medications. She was restricted to toe-touch weight bearing on the right lower extremity for 6 weeks post-operatively. A CPM was initiated on POD #1 with a ROM from 0 to 90°. X-rays were obtained prior to leaving the hospital (immediate postoperative X-rays).

She returned to the clinic at 2 weeks for suture removal and was noted to have excellent pain relief. At 6 weeks post-op, the patient was advanced to partial weight bearing with the use of a single crutch and allowed to advance to weight bearing as tolerated over the next month. At 4 months she was noted to have some lateral hip pain and underwent screw removal. At final follow-up, 2 years after the index surgery, she is doing very well. She runs approximately 15 min per day without any significant pain. Her X-rays show a healed osteonecrotic segment of femoral head without any additional collapse. The lateral X-ray at 2 years shows the area of harvest and the healing of the grafts quite nicely. She was very pleased with the results and we will plan to see her back in 5 years from the initial surgical date.

Immediate post-operative X-rays:

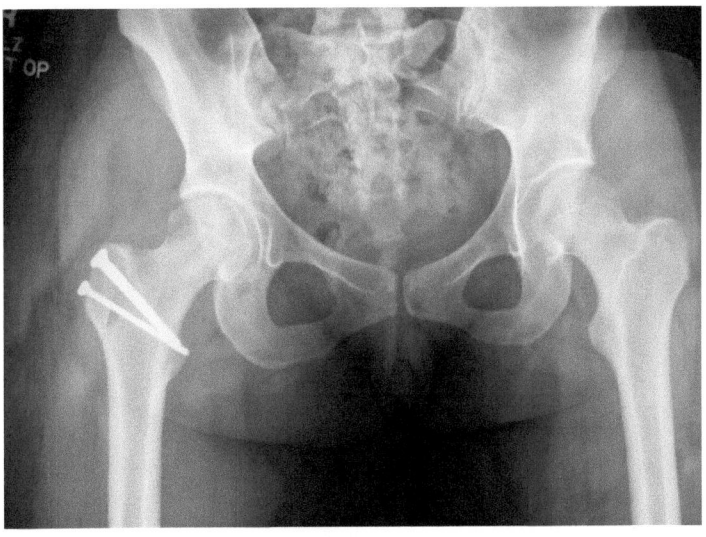

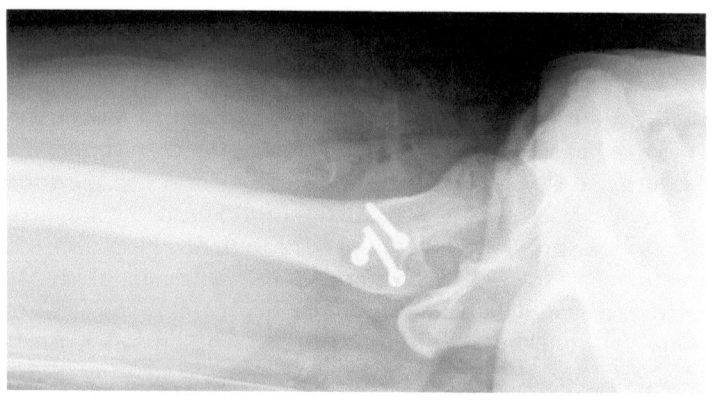

Five months post-operative:

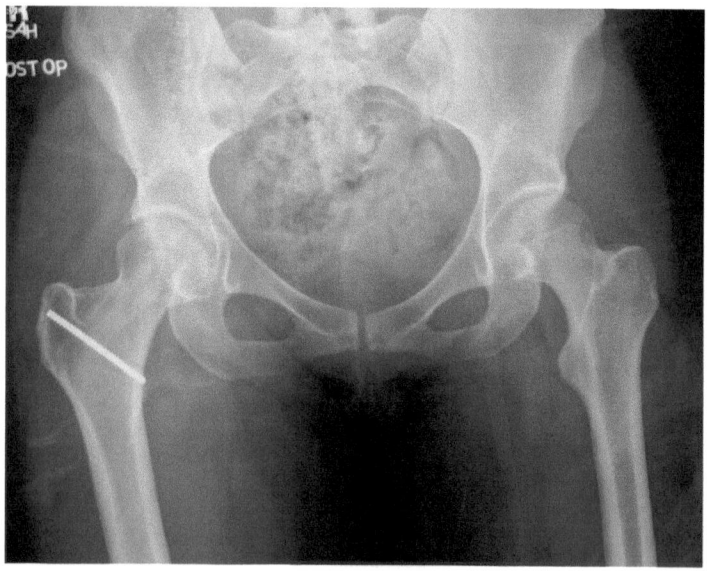

Two-year post-operative X-rays:

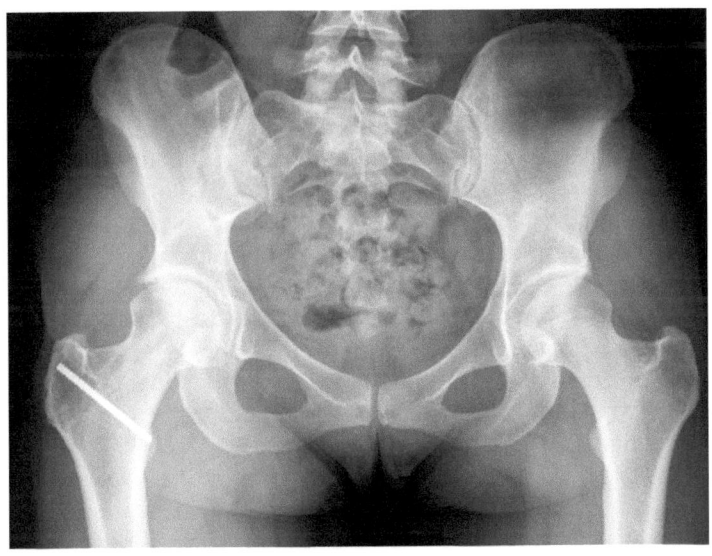

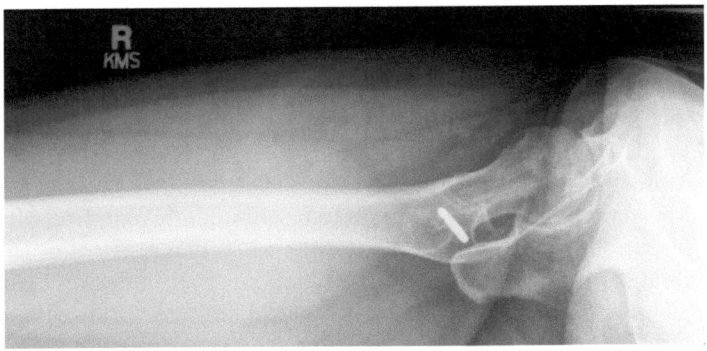

Literature Review

There have been very few studies examining patients treated with osteochondral autografts for femoral head lesions. One of the earliest studies of autograft transplantation of the femoral head was conducted by Meyers et al. [1]. The study identifies three case reports of patients that underwent a Gibson approach to the femoral head; the cartilage overlying the necrotic lesion was sharply incised and elevated around three fourths of the lytic lesion. The necrotic bone was resected and packed with autologous iliac crest bone graft and the flap was then closed over the bone graft. Two of the three patients noted marked improvement in pain and function. The other patient continued to have weight-bearing pain and was eventually converted to a total hip arthroplasty at 6 months postoperatively.

More recently there have been a few case reports on patients that underwent osteochondral autograft transplantation to the femoral head utilizing a surgical hip dislocation. The first study is a case report of a 36-year-old male with bilateral femoral AVN [2]. An anterolateral approach was utilized to access the femoral head. A large AVN lesion was noted on the femoral head and the cartilage and necrotic bone was removed. Three osteochondral autograft bone plugs were obtained from the non-weight-bearing inferolateral aspect of the femoral head. These grafts were inserted in to the AVN defect in a mosaicplasty fashion similar to our case. The patient was followed for 66 months and noted to be completely pain-free with no evidence of femoral head collapse radiographically. The final study is a case report of two patients that underwent surgical hip dislocation and osteochondral autograft transplantation from the knee in one and from the inferolateral femoral head in the other patient to the necrotic lesion of the femoral head [3]. Both patients had MRIs performed which showed graft incorporation of the femoral head osteochondral autograft and both were able to return to an active lifestyle postoperatively. There have been only retrospective case reports in the literature to date; however, these case reports show promising results at short- to mid-term follow-up.

Clinical Pearls and Pitfalls

- Dissection in between the piriformis and minimus will avoid injury to the anastomotic branch between the deep branch of the medial femoral circumflex and the inferior gluteal vessels, occasionally the sole blood supply to the femoral head.
- The trochanteric osteotomy should be at least 15 mm thick to avoid fracture with fixation.
- While performing the Z-plasty of the capsulotomy, care should be utilized to avoid damaging the labrum and femoral head articular cartilage.
- Obtain osteochondral autograft from the non-weight-bearing area of the femoral head.
- Ensure that the osteochondral autograft is recessed at the level of the femoral head articular cartilage.
- Large osteonecrotic defects are unlikely treatable with an osteochondral autograft transplant and may require an allograft or joint replacement (in this case we were unable to achieve complete excision of the damaged cartilage, we decided to only graft the most weight-bearing zone, obtaining good results). Mapping on the cartilage defect will allow planning for size of osteochondral plugs. Obtaining more than 3 plugs from the inferior and medial aspect of the femoral head is unlikely.
- Patient selection is critical: young patients with minor areas of segmental collapse with cartilage degeneration may benefit from this procedure; this should only be done in patients where trauma is suspected as the risk factor that has led to the osteonecrosis. In secondary cases, this treatment is unlikely to prevent progression of the disease.
- If, at the time of surgery, the area of collapse demonstrates relatively well-preserved articular cartilage, a trapdoor procedure with elevation of the cartilage and bone grafting may be a better option over osteochondral autograft.

References

1. Meyers MH, et al. Fresh autogenous grafts and osteochondral allografts for the treatment of segmental collapse in osteonecrosis of the hip. Clin Orthop Relat Res. 1983;174:107–12.
2. Sotereanos NG, et al. Autogenous osteochondral transfer in the femoral head after osteonecrosis. Orthopedics. 2008;31(2):177.
3. Nam D, et al. Traumatic osteochondral injury of the femoral head treated by mosaicplasty: a report of two cases. HSS J. 2010;6(2):228–34.

Chapter 15
Long-Term Result of Hip Decompression and Vascularized Fibula for Steinberg Stage IV AVN

Vasili Karas, Patrick Millikan, and Samuel Wellman

Case Presentation

The patient is a 28-year-old male who was involved in a motor vehicle accident 1 year prior to presentation. Due to cerebrospinal trauma, the patient required high-dose corticosteroids at the time of his injury. He presented with increasing bilateral groin pain, worse with weight bearing, and is also troublesome at night. Despite attempts at activity modification and oral anti-inflammatory medications, his pain persisted and affected his activities of daily living.

V. Karas, MD • P. Millikan, MD • S. Wellman, MD (✉)
Duke University Medical Center and Durham VA Medical Center, Durham, NC, Box 3447, 27710, USA
e-mail: Samuel.Wellman@duke.edu

R.J. Sierra (ed.), *Osteonecrosis of the Femoral Head*,
DOI 10.1007/978-3-319-50664-7_15,
© Mayo Foundation for Medical Education and Research 2017

A focused physical examination of the lower extremities revealed full extension and external rotation at the hip bilaterally. He was unable to exceed 0 of internal rotation or adduction due to pain. His gait was antalgic and favored the right hip. His knee ankle and foot exam were unremarkable. He was neurovascularly intact with full strength throughout the lower extremities bilaterally. AP and frog leg lateral radiographs revealed bilateral subchondral sclerosis within the femoral head with preserved joint space. The femoral head showed evidence of flattening on the right (Fig. 15.1a, b). The patient felt his pain was debilitating and causing poor quality of life. After lengthy discussion, he requested surgical intervention with preservation of his native hip if possible.

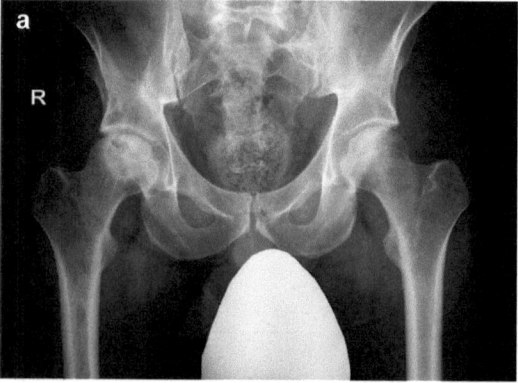

FIGURE 15.1 Anterior-posterior pelvis (**a**), and bilateral hip frog leg lateral (**b**) radiographs of a 28-year-old patient with bilateral hip pain on presentation. The femoral head shows evidence of flattening on the right and a lesion without collapse on the left

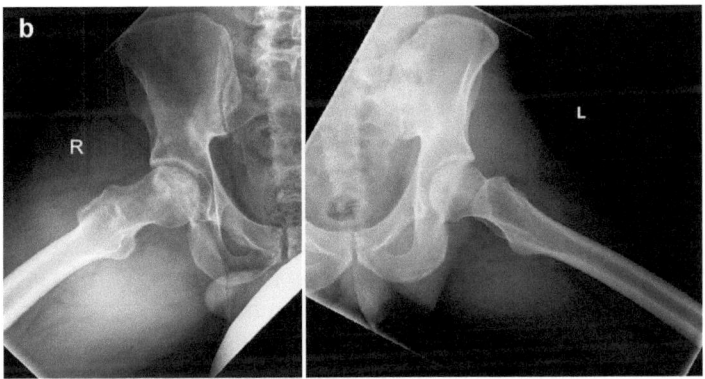

FIGURE 15.1 (continued)

Diagnosis/Assessment

The patient's history, physical examination, and radiographic studies were consistent with osteonecrosis of the femoral head (ONFH). Flattening and/or collapse on imaging with preservation of joint space, as in this patient's case, is classified as Steinberg stage IV ONFH. Given the patient's age and preserved joint space with approximately 1 mm of collapse, he was a candidate for a hip-preserving operation or a total hip arthroplasty (THA).

Management

The patient elected to undergo free vascularized fibular graft of the right hip as pain from the right was the most debilitating. Both total hip arthroplasty and free vascularized fibular graft (FVFG) were discussed as options for the patient. He elected to proceed with FVFG, citing the desire to preserve his native hip and delay arthroplasty as long as possible. The patient was then taken to the operating room where a free vascularized fibular graft was harvested and subsequently implanted into the femoral neck and head after core decompression and local bone grafting. This was performed as described by Aldridge et al. [1]. The technique consists of harvesting of the fibula and preparation of the graft site, either by two teams in concert or by a single team in a stepwise fashion. The patient is placed in the lateral decubitus position, and the hip is approached via an anterolateral incision [2]. The fascia lata is incised longitudinally, extending proximally between the gluteus maximus and tensor fascia lata, exposing the proximolateral femur. Deep dissection continues deep to the abductors and rectus femoris, permitting the dissection of the donor vessels, which are usually the ascending branches of the lateral femoral circumflex artery and its accompanying veins [3]. A Steinmann pin is inserted from the lateral femur through the neck into the femoral head lesion under fluoroscopic guidance. Sequential reamers are introduced over the pin, and reaming continues until a tunnel of sufficient diameter to allow placement of the fibula strut is achieved, with reaming continuing proximally to within about 5 mm from the articular surface of the femoral head. Remaining necrotic bone is then removed with a curette while using fluoroscopy to evaluate the borders of the lesion. Contrast dye can be injected into the tunnel to further appreciate its characteristics [4]. Viable cancellous reamings and autograft harvested from the greater trochanter are packed into the tunnel once the necrotic bone is removed.

The ipsilateral fibula is approached via a lateral incision, described by Judet [5]. The peroneal vessel pedicle is identified and freed from surrounding soft tissue. Proximal and distal osteotomies are performed, and the graft is freed. The final steps of this portion of the case can be delayed if needed until the femur is prepared to accept the graft [1].

Once the fibula is prepared and the tunnel is complete, the graft can be released from the donor site and introduced into the femoral tunnel (Fig. 15.2b). The graft is placed such that the pedicle is unimpeded and patent, and so the fibular graft is abutting the subchondral plate and newly introduced cancellous graft (Fig. 15.3a). The graft is then secured with a Kirschner wire, and the arterial and venous anastomoses are

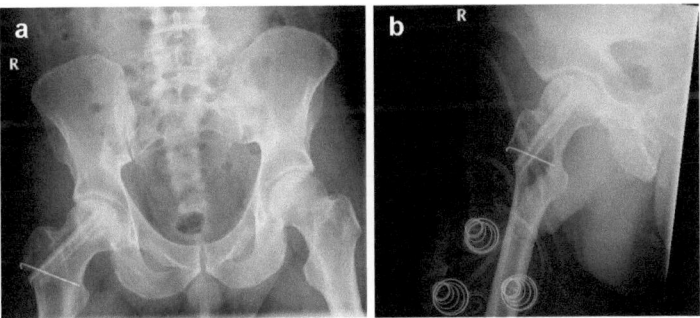

FIGURE 15.2 Anterior-posterior pelvis (**a**) and frog leg lateral (**b**) of the left hip on postoperative day one after free vascularized fibular graft

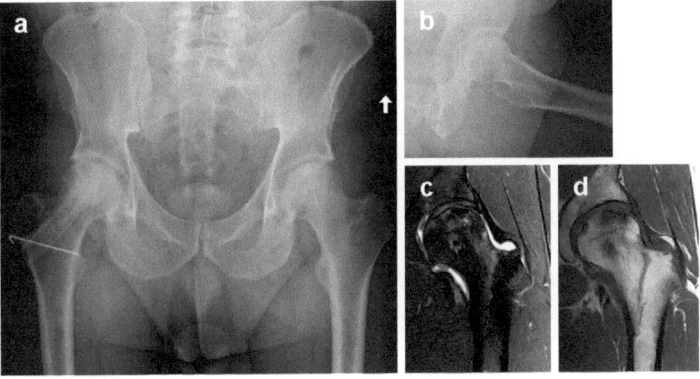

FIGURE 15.3 Anterior-posterior pelvis radiograph (**a**) and frog leg lateral of the left hip (**b**) of the, now, 30-year-old patient 2 years status post right free vascularized fibular graft. At the time of this radiograph, the patient presents with increased pain and difficulty weight bearing on the left hip. An MRI was obtained at the time. Coronal T2 (**c**) and T1 (**d**) demonstrate AVN and flattening of central superior femoral head

performed with the aid of microscopy. Blood flow into the graft is confirmed by seeing endosteal bleeding inside the fibular canal (Fig. 15.2c) [5]. Of note, there was a moderate amount of avascular bone removed from the femoral head, and after anastomosis, intraosseous bleeding was noted at the base of the fibula. Figure 15.2a, b demonstrates immediate postoperative radiographs of the left hip.

Outcome

The patient convalesced as expected. At 1 year from surgery, he stated minimal pain on the right and required no ambulatory aid. In general, patients are made non-weight bearing for the first 6 weeks after surgery. They are then slowly progressed to full weight bearing over another 6 weeks with return to weight bearing as tolerated at 3 months postoperatively. At 2 years postoperatively, the patient presented with desire to undergo the same procedure on the left hip. Radiographs and magnetic resonance imaging of the left hip demonstrated flattening and ONFH with preserved joint space (Fig. 15.3a–d). Of note, this was less severe than the right. The patient underwent the procedure once more on the contralateral side uneventfully.

At most recent follow-up, the patient was 5 years from FVFG on the right and 3 years from surgery on the left. Unfortunately, his right hip has begun increasingly painful, requiring the use of a cane (Fig. 15.4). His most recent imaging demonstrated increased sclerosis of the right femoral head as well as lateral joint space narrowing. There was also evidence of 1–2 mm of increased collapse seen between the 1-year follow-up and 2-year follow-up radiographs (Fig. 15.5a–c).

Due to his symptoms, the patient elected to undergo right total hip arthroplasty 5 years after his initial FVFG. Surgery was recently performed. An AP pelvis radiograph immediately postoperatively is shown in Fig. 15.6. Of note, he continues to have minimal pain and good function of the left hip. Given the overall relief of pain for 5 years, the patient was relatively happy with the result of the hip-preserving technique.

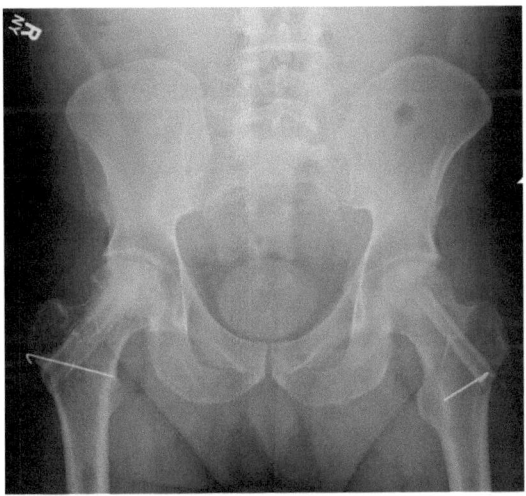

FIGURE 15.4 Anterior-posterior pelvis radiograph at 3 months post-operatively from left and 3 years postoperatively from right free vascularized fibular graft. At the time of this radiograph, the patient presents with increased pain. The joint space on the right is decreased laterally and there is interval presence of subchondral sclerosis and femoral head collapse

Literature Review

The patient's history, physical, and images are consistent with osteonecrosis of the femoral head (ONFH). As always, a thorough history and physical is vital. This may reveal the presence of risk factors for ONFH, such as former steroid use, alcohol abuse, or clotting disorders [7, 8]. Patients with early stages this of disease are often asymptomatic. When the condition becomes painful, most patients will complain of deep pain within the groin. Pain is sometimes referred to the ipsilateral buttock or knee. On physical exam, patients often exhibit painful internal rotation. Limited internal rotation may be suggestive of collapse of the femoral head [4].

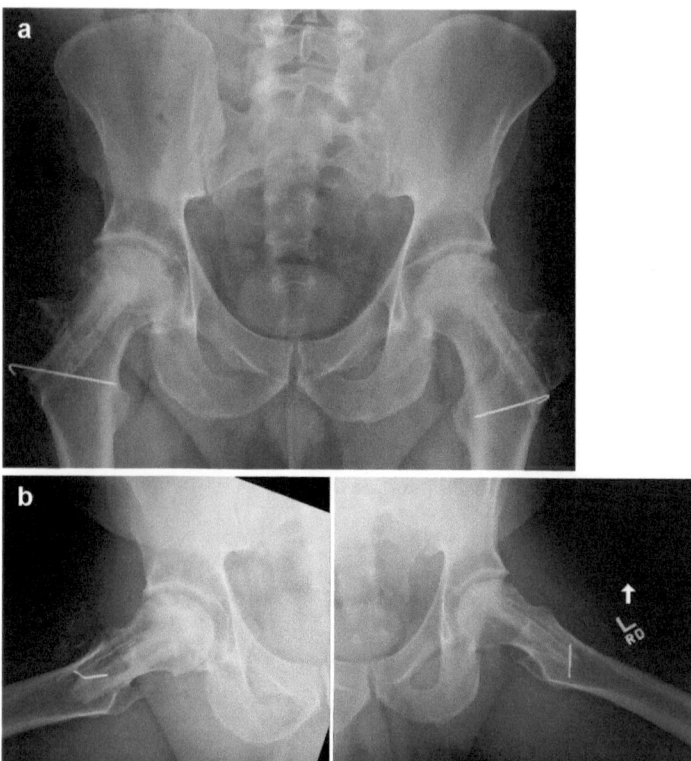

FIGURE 15.5 Anterior-posterior pelvis radiograph (**a**) and bilateral frog leg lateral (**b**) of the patient 5 years postoperatively on the right and 3 years postoperatively on the left from free vascularized fibular graft. At the time of these radiographs, the patient presents with increase pain on the right with weight bearing and requests total hip arthroplasty. The left hip also shows a segment of collapse and is intermittently painful but does not impede function

Diagnosis and staging of ONFH is made using plain films and MRI. Though plain films can be negative in early stages, sclerotic or cystic changes of the femoral often manifest quickly. MRI is 99% sensitive and specific for diagnosis of ONFH [8]. Multiple staging systems exist for evaluating

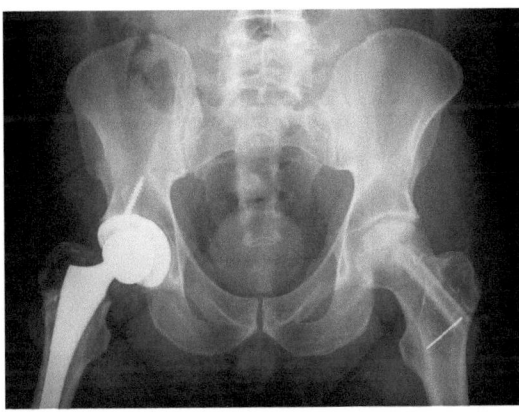

FIGURE 15.6 Anterior-posterior pelvis radiograph immediately post-operatively after right total hip replacement. Left hip 3.5 years status post FVFG

ONFH. The Steinberg classification is one such system. Staging in the Steinberg classification focuses on patient symptoms and radiographic findings. In Steinberg stage IV, the patient is symptomatic. The shape of the femoral head has been affected by the death of subchondral bone, causing flattening or collapse of the dome. However, at this stage, the acetabulum has yet to become involved [9].

Steinberg stage IV is further separated into three substages, IVA, IVB, and IVC. These substages identify the percentage of articular surface collapsed and the extent of the damage. In stage IVA, less than 15% of the articular surface is involved, with less than 2 mm of articular step-off. In IVB, 15–30% is involved, with 2–4 mm of step-off. In IVC, greater than 30% is collapsed [9].

Surgical treatment of patients with ONFH varies widely, depending on the severity of disease. For stage IV lesions, treatment options consist of core decompression although not recommended currently, vascularized grafting, or arthroplasty.

Core decompression (CD) involves the removal of necrotic subchondral bone by drilling into the femoral head via the neck. This can be performed via one large tract, or multiple smaller tracts. The goal is to depressurize the necrotic subchondral bone and introduce bleeding into previously avascular tissue. Decompression can be supplemented with bone graft, as well as other additives, discussed later [6].

Mont et al. in 1998 reviewed 52 patients with 68 hips treated with CD for ONFH, with a goal of discovering usable prognostic indicators for postoperative survivorship. Patients had a mean follow-up of 12 years after CD. Of the 44 hips classified as Steinberg stage III, 41% (18 hips) underwent THA by 12 years. This varied significantly from the stage IV group, who experienced a 92% (22/24 hips) conversion rate. The authors concluded that the best predictor of a satisfactory outcome for patients with ONFH included stage III disease or less [6].

These results were reiterated by Steinberg et al. in 2001, who prospectively studied 406 hips in 285 patients, all treated by one surgeon using core decompression (CD) with supplemental bone grafting. Harris hip score, radiographic progression, and need for conversional to total hip arthroplasty (THA) were evaluated. These results were compared to a control group of 55 hips in 39 patients who were treated nonoperatively. All patients underwent a minimum 2-year follow-up [10].

Of 92 hips evaluated as Steinberg stage IV, 49% (45 hips) treated with CD were converted THA at 2 years. This varied significantly from the 90% conversion rate within the control group. Percent conversion was slightly lower in pre-collapse patients (Steinberg III) treated with CD, with 3 of 13 (23%) requiring conversion, versus 82% of the control group. Steinberg stage I and II only saw a combined 28% conversion rate at 2 years, though this was mostly in patients with lesions involving >15% of the articular surface. Significant differences in outcome scores were seen in operative patients with minor (stages I and II) lesions. The authors concluded that surgical treatment via CD for ONFH was beneficial in the delay of THA, especially in pre-collapse (Steinberg I, II, and III) patients [10].

Marker et al. in 2008 performed a literature review to determine if outcomes of patients undergoing CD have improved over time. They compared results in the literature, as well as their own cohort of 79 hips, both before and after 1992. They discovered a decrease in additional surgeries, as well as an increase in radiographic success in patients treated after 1992. However, they noted that fewer patients were treated with preoperative lesions classified as Ficat III (Steinberg stage IV) as time progressed. The best overall results were seen in patients with Ficat stage I lesions. This suggests that the improvement in patient outcomes is likely due to patient selection, as patients with more advanced lesions were treated with other procedures [12].

A criticism of the theory behind CD states that, since few progenitor cells exist within the remaining bone of the avascular femoral head, core decompression and bone grafting alone should not be expected to encourage healing of bone. Hernigou et al. in 2015 performed a literature review to determine the "state of the art" in the addition of supplemental materials during CD and bone grafting for ONFH. Overall, patients experienced improved outcomes when the CD was supplemented with either autologous bone marrow cells or mesenchymal stem cells, both autologous and allogenic. Importantly, there were no adverse events associated with the treatments, suggesting supplementation of this procedure may represent a safe, beneficial addition [13].

Free vascularized fibular graft (FVFG) involves the harvest and free transfer of a vascularized fibular graft to the prepared femoral head in a patient with ONFH. The technique was developed simultaneously at several institutions, with the rise of operative microscopy. The fibula is prepared and harvested from the ipsilateral leg with the peroneal vessel pedicle intact. Meanwhile, the femoral head is prepared and reamed, similar to the process of CD. The fibula is then introduced as a vascularized autograft that provided support and blood supply to the subchondral bone. If there is any collapse, a custom fluted bone tamp specific to the procedure both introduces autologous bone and elevates the collapsed subchondral bone.

Berend et al. in 2003 investigated the role of FVFG in the treatment of post-collapse ONFH [14]. He retrospectively reviewed the treatment of 188 patients (224 hips), with average follow-up of 4.3 years. Failure of graft was defined as conversion to THA. At 5 years, 64% of hips survived after FVFG. The authors concluded that risk for failure was increased in patients with idiopathic ONFH or disease associated with alcohol abuse and trauma. Interestingly, joint survival was not significantly related to size of the lesion, though there was an increased relative risk for THA with larger lesion size with simultaneous collapse.

With the complex nature of FVFG, it becomes important to evaluate the longevity of the procedure. Yoo et al. in 2008 retrospectively reviewed 110 patients (124 hips) with a minimum follow-up of 10 years (average of 13.9 years) [15]. For hips with Ficat III lesions, 39 out of 65 (60%) had improved or unchanged radiographs. At 10 years, 10.5% (13/135) hips had undergone THA. Eward et al. examined a similar question in 2011. They performed a retrospective review of 61 patients (65 hips) who underwent FVFG for pre-collapse ONFH, with a minimum follow-up of 10.5 years. They found 75% (65 hips) had surviving grafts at 10 years. Twenty-six hips (40%) underwent THA at a mean of 8 years after FVFG. The authors concluded that FVFG still served an important role in the treatment of ONFH in patients under 50 years of age with pre-collapse osteonecrosis of the femoral head [16].

FVFG is not without complications. Aldridge et al. in 2007 reviewed 2600 patients who underwent FVFG between 1979 and 2006. The complication rate was relatively low, but included significant incidents. These include subtrochanteric fracture (1%), surgical site infection (0.03%), great toe plantarflexion contracture (3%), and ankle pain (10%) [4]. Another criticism of FVFG is the cost. Careful scrutiny has found FVFG to be cost-effective, despite the intricate surgery and postoperative course [17].

A comparison of FVFG and CD must be performed when determining the best treatment path for the patient with ONFH. This decision has been examined within the literature.

Trousdale in 1997 prospectively compared the outcomes of 39 hips in 34 patients with Ficat II and III ONFH. Twenty patients underwent FVFG, while 19 underwent core decompression. Imaging was assessed at 2 years postoperatively, with failure being defined as conversion to THA for "incapacitating pain." Patients who underwent FVFG have a failure rate of 20% at 2 years, significantly lower that of the CD group. Interestingly, all of the failures within the FVFG group were patients with Ficat stage III disease, while patients with Ficat stage I/II disease had no failure [11].

When discussing the post-collapse patient specifically, a comparison of techniques becomes more black and white. Beaule et al. examined the treatment of Ficat stage III and IV disease [18]. He performed a literature review, summarizing the outcomes and treatment strategies for this complex population. His conclusions stated that, though CD can produced good outcomes in patients with pre-collapse disease, the procedure has "no role" in the treatment of patients after femoral head collapse. Despite the better results achieved by FVFG, he states that the high complication rate paired with high rates of conversion to THA proves it is not a perfect solution.

Total hip arthroplasty (THA) is a viable treatment option in ONFH, especially in the presence of collapse. As materials and techniques continue to advance, many consider THA the first-line treatment, even for the young patient. Hungerford et al. in 2007 stated that the advancement in technique, as well as new bearing surfaces, has altered the "save-at-all-costs paradigm." The author argues that these advances should make certain high-cost, low-success operations (such as femoral osteotomy and FVFG) obsolete, especially in patients with collapse of the articulating surface [19].

Though the advancements in THA make it an enticing consideration in treatment of ONFH, recent studies suggest an increased complication rate among this patient population. Yang et al. in 2015 reviewed the Medicare database to evaluate the outcomes of ONFH patients treated with THA [20]. The author discovered an increased postoperative complication rate, including component loosening, osteolysis, dislocation, as well as renal and respiratory issues. Stavrakis et al. in 2015 reviewed the hospital admissions in THA patients in California from 1995 to 2010 [21]. He then compared the postoperative course of patients with concomitant history of ONFH versus those without. He discovered a significantly increased risk of readmission and sepsis in patients with THA secondary to ONFH. This data suggest that, despite the numerous benefits when treating ONFH with THA, the patient population may be more prone to the known complications of this surgery. On the contrary, Berend et al. demonstrated a femoral stem revision rate in total hip arthroplasty after FVFG of 7.4% at 9-year follow-up, which is similar to that of the femoral stem revision rate in primary surgery [22].

THA as the primary procedure for ONFH is a considerably more viable option today than previous years. Concerns for short- to midterm osteolysis and need for revision after total hip arthroplasty are lower today, with optimized fixation and highly cross-linked polyethylene liners.

Clinical Pearls and Pitfalls

- Core decompression (CD) does not have a real roll in patients with post-collapse osteonecrosis of the femoral head (ONFH). Free vascularized fibular graft should be considered in this population, though poorer outcomes have been reported when compared to pre-collapse patients. Finally, total hip arthroplasty (THA) can also be contemplated, though this has been historically avoided in young patients.
- When considering THA, consider FVFG. In the young patient, THA may be limiting and necessitate high likelihood of repeat surgery in the future. In the pre-collapse patient, vascularized grafting can help delay THA and may provide definitive relief of symptoms.

- FVFG is not perfect. Though some patients have excellent long-term results, others do not. Realistic outcomes after FVFG in Steinberg IV hips are 65% survival at 5 years. Reported complication rates are as high as 25% including contracture of the flexor hallucis longus, ankle pain, proximal femoral fracture, and infection.
- Careful consideration of the vessels during microsurgical anastomosis is vital to success, specifically, attempting to match the caliber of the donor vessel to that of the lateral circumflex branch. Furthermore, adequate pedicle length (a minimum of 4 cm) at time of fibular harvest allows for a tension-free anastomosis, decreasing postoperative leaking and ultimate failure.
- Stripping of the pedicle during insertion of the graft is a potential error. This is avoided by securing the pedicle to the end of the fibular graft, often with a single suture. Adequate placement of the fibular graft into the subchondral bone is required for appropriate structural support. A vascular clip can be placed on the superior end of the graft, allowing the use of fluoroscopic imaging to guarantee the appropriate placement of the fibula.

References

1. Aldridge 3rd JM, Berend KR, Gunneson EE, Urbaniak JR. Free vascularized fibular grafting for the treatment of postcollapse osteonecrosis of the femoral head. Surgical technique. J Bone Joint Surg Am. 2004;86-A(Suppl 1):87–101.
2. Marchant Jr MH, Zura RD, Urbaniak JR, Aldridge 3rd JM. Hip incision planning for free vascularized fibular grafting of the proximal femur: a handy tip. J Surg Orthop Adv. 2007;16:204–6.
3. Soucacos PN, Beris AE, Malizos K, Koropilias A, Zalavras H, Dailiana Z. Treatment of avascular necrosis of the femoral head

with vascularized fibular transplant. Clin Orthop Relat Res. 2001;386:120–30.

4. Aldridge III JM, Urbaniak JR. Avascular necrosis of the femoral head: role of vascularized bone grafts. Orthop Clin North Am. 2007;38:13–22.

5. Judet H, Judet J, Gilbert A. Vascular microsurgery in orthopaedics. Int Orthop. 1981;5:61–8.

6. Mont MA, Etienne G, Ragland PS. Outcome of nonvascularized bone grafting for osteonecrosis of the femoral head. Clin Orthop Relat Res. 2003;417:84–92.

7. Hernigou P, Bachir D, Galacteros F. The natural history of symptomatic osteonecrosis in adults with sickle-cell disease. J Bone Joint Surg. 2003;85:500–4.

8. Zalavras CG, Lieberman JR. Osteonecrosis of the femoral head: evaluation and treatment. J Am Acad Orthop Surg. 2014;22:455–64.

9. Lieberman JR, Berry DJ, Mont MA, et al. Osteonecrosis of the hip: management in the 21st century. Instr Course Lect. 2003;52:337–55.

10. Steinberg ME, Larcom PG, Strafford B, et al. Core decompression with bone grafting for osteonecrosis of the femoral head. Clin Orthop. 2001;386:71–8.

11. Trousdale RT. Vascularized free fibula graft vs core decompression. Orthopedics. 1997;20(4):359.

12. Marker DR, Seyler TM, Ulrich SD, Srivastava S, Mont MA. Do modern techniques improve core decompression outcomes for hip osteonecrosis? Clin Orthop. 2008;466:1093–103.

13. Hernigou P, Flouzat-Lachaniette C, Delambre J, et al. Osteonecrosis repair with bone marrow cell therapies: state of the clinical art. Bone. 2015;70:102–9.

14. Berend KR, Gunneson EE, Urbaniak JR. Free vascularized fibular grafting for the treatment of postcollapse osteonecrosis of the femoral head. J Bone Joint Surg Am. 2003;85-A:987–93.

15. Yoo MC, Kim KI, Hahn CS, Parvizi J. Long-term followup of vascularized fibular grafting for femoral head necrosis. Clin Orthop Relat Res. 2008;466:1133–40.

16. Eward WC, Rineer CA, Urbaniak JR, Richard MJ, Ruch DS. The vascularized fibular graft in precollapse osteonecrosis: is long-term hip preservation possible? Clin Orthop Relat Res. 2012;470:2819–26.

17. Watters TS, Browne JA, Orlando LA, Wellman SS, Urbaniak JR, Bolognesi MP. Cost-effectiveness analysis of free vascularized

fibular grafting for osteonecrosis of the femoral head. J Surg Orthop Adv. 2011;20:158–67.

18. Beaule PE, Amstutz HC. Management of Ficat stage III and IV osteonecrosis of the hip. J Am Acad Orthop Surg. 2004;12:96–105.

19. Hungerford DS. Treatment of osteonecrosis of the femoral head: everything's new. J Arthroplasty. 2007;22:91–4.

20. Yang S, Halim AY, Werner BC, Gwathmey FW, Cui Q. Does osteonecrosis of the femoral head increase surgical and medical complication rates after total hip arthroplasty? A comprehensive analysis in the United States. Hip Int. 2015;25:237–44.

21. Stavrakis A, SooHoo N, Lieberman J. A comparison of the incidence of complications following total hip arthroplasty in patients with or without osteonecrosis. J Arthroplasty. 2015;30:114–7.

22. Berend KR, Gunneson E, Urbaniak JR, Vail TP. Hip arthroplasty after failed free vascularized fibular grafting for osteonecrosis in young patients. J Arthroplasty. 2003;18:411–9.

Chapter 16
Bone Grafting Pedicled with Femoral Quadratus for Alcohol-Induced Osteonecrosis of the Femoral Head

Yisheng Wang

Case Presentation

A 31-year-old male patient bilateral alcohol-induced ONFH for 2 years. He had a 10-year drinking history with drinking 500 cc or more of alcohol daily. On physical examination at clinic, the patient had hip pain and slight limp. He had limited mobility of the hip and a positive "Patrick's test." On the radiographic films and MRI findings, the signs of ONFH were clearly visible. According to the classification system of the Association Research Circulation Osseous (ARCO), the right femoral head was in stage II-B and the left side was in stage II-C. The patient was treated by the bone grafting

Y. Wang, MD, PhD
Department of Orthopaedic Surgery, 1st Affiliated Hospital of Zhengzhou University, Zhengzhou, Henan province, China
e-mail: wangyisheng@zzu.edu.cn

R.J. Sierra (ed.), *Osteonecrosis of the Femoral Head*,
DOI 10.1007/978-3-319-50664-7_16,
© Mayo Foundation for Medical Education and Research 2017

pedicled with femoral quadratus for the left femoral head and the right 10 days later. The postoperative X-ray films showed thoroughly removed necrotic bone, sufficient grafting bone, and well strut position of grafting bone column in the femoral heads.

Diagnosis/Assessment

This younger patient's history, physical examination, and radiographic findings are consistent with the diagnosis of alcohol-induced ONFH and in stages of pre-collapse. To avoid misdiagnosis we should also pay attention to the differential diagnosis with other diseases such as bone marrow edema, synovial hernia, tumor, tuberculosis, osteoarthritis, and hip dysplasia.

The treatment of ONFH should be individualized based on the patient's age, size and shape of the osteonecrosis, and risk or presence of collapse. Optimal outcome can only be achieved by good understanding of treatment principles and choosing proper treatment methods for each stage of ONFH. Joint preservation should be preferred in young patients. This technique is best when performed for ONFH in stages of pre-collapse.

Management

The surgical steps for the bone grafting pedicled with femoral quadratus are present in schematic diagram (Fig. 16.1).

1. Approach and incision: Under general anesthesia with endotracheal intubation, the operation was performed with the patient in a lateral decubitus position. The Moore approach (posterior incision) is adopted.
2. Obtain grafting bone pedicled with femoral quadratus, cortical bone strips, and cancellous bone pellets and flakes: Expose the external rotator muscles of hip and carefully

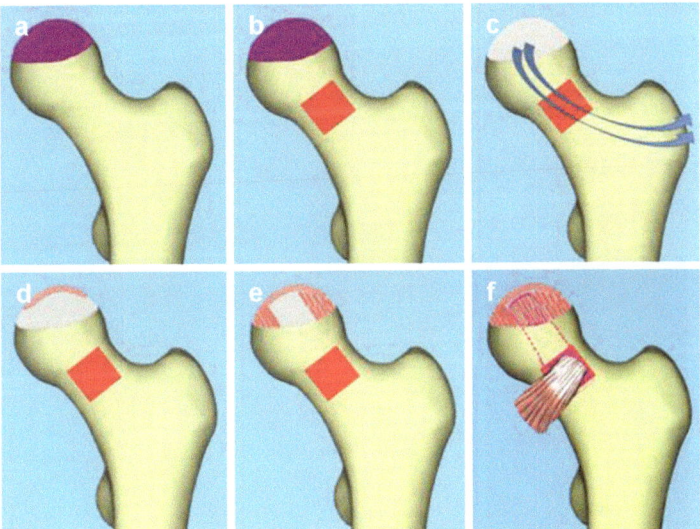

FIGURE 16.1 Diagram of bone grafting pedicled with femoral quadratus. (**a**) ONFH. (**b**) A fenestration groove is made below the cartilage edge of the femoral head at the posterior side of the femoral neck. (**c**) Thoroughly removed necrotic bone. (**d**) The cancellous bone balls and flakes are put onto the inner surface of cartilage of the cavity. (**e**) The many cancellous bone flake and matchstick cortical bone strips were planted on inner walls of the empty cavity in the femoral head and pressed solid. A big and long straight passage in the center of the femoral head is reserved, which connected with the fenestration of femoral neck. (**f**) The graft bone column pedicled with femoral quadratus is implanted into the straight passage in the center of the femoral head and inserted into the fenestration groove at the distal side

separate the upper and lower edges of the femoral quadratus, and cut off the attachment points of obturator and gemellus muscle on the femur. After the posterior intertrochanteric area with the insertion of the femoral quadratus is identified, a rectangular bone block pedicled with the femoral quadratus is obtained using an osteotome. Its length should be 3.5–5.0 cm, width of 1.4–2.0 cm, and thickness of 1.0–2.0 cm (Fig. 16.2a, b). The largest bone block can be used it up to 2.0 × 2.0 × 5.0 cm. In addition,

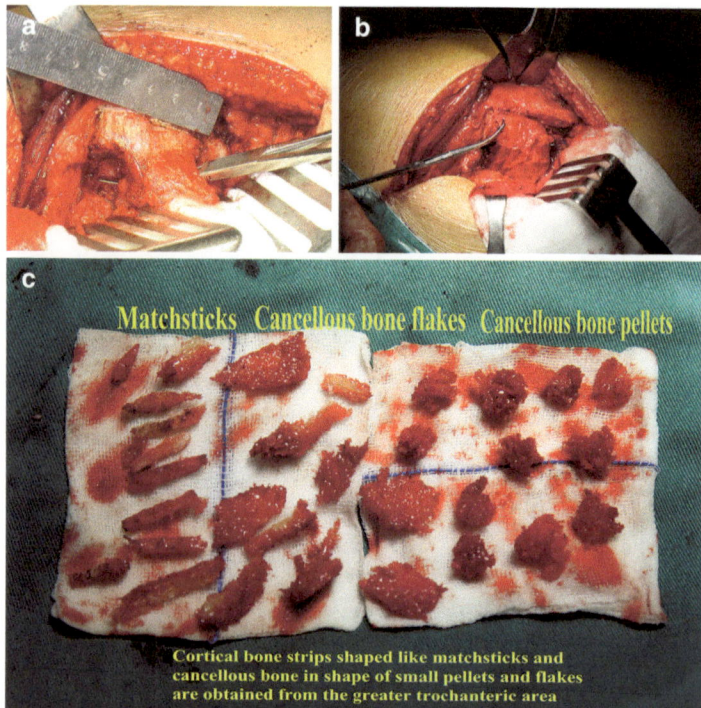

FIGURE 16.2 (**a**, **b**) Obtain graft bone pedicled with femoral quadra-tus. (**c**) Cortical bone strips shaped like matchsticks and cancellous bone in shape of small pellets and flakes

cortical bone strips shaped like matchsticks and cancellous bone in shape of small pellets and flakes are obtained from the greater trochanteric area (Fig. 16.2c).

3. Thoroughly remove necrotic bone: The posterior part of joint capsule is resected. A fenestration groove in size of 1.4 × 1.4 cm is made below the cartilage edge of the femo-ral head at the posterior side of the femoral neck (Fig. 16.3a). Through this window, the necrotic bone is thoroughly removed until the inner surface of cartilage by using osteotome, curette, or burr (Fig. 16.3b, c). The necrotic

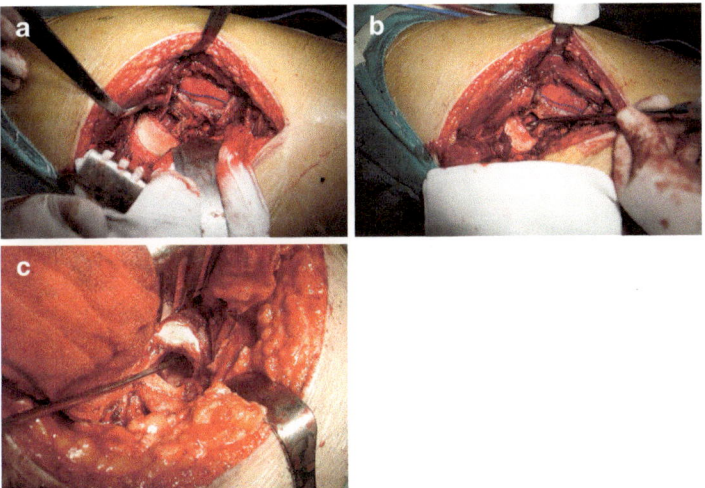

FIGURE 16.3 Thoroughly remove necrotic bone. (**a**) A window is made below the cartilage edge of the femoral head at the posterior side of the femoral neck. (**b, c**) Thoroughly remove necrotic bone up to the inner surface of cartilage of the necrotic bone area by using an osteotome, curette, or burr

area is usually located in the superior and anterior lateral region in the femoral head and can be seen clearly when performing this posterior approach. Care should be taken not to cut through or scratch and perforate the cartilage layer. The depth of the empty cavity usually measures around 3.5 cm.

4. Bone grafting:

After thoroughly removing the necrotic bone, the necrotic region becomes a large empty cavity within the femoral head, like a vacant shell. First, cancellous bone pellets and flakes are impacted tightly into the inner surface of cartilage of the cavity. The thickness of accumulated cancellous bone is about 5 mm (Fig. 16.4a1, a2). Second, more cancellous bone flakes and matchstick-shaped cortical bone strips are planted onto the around

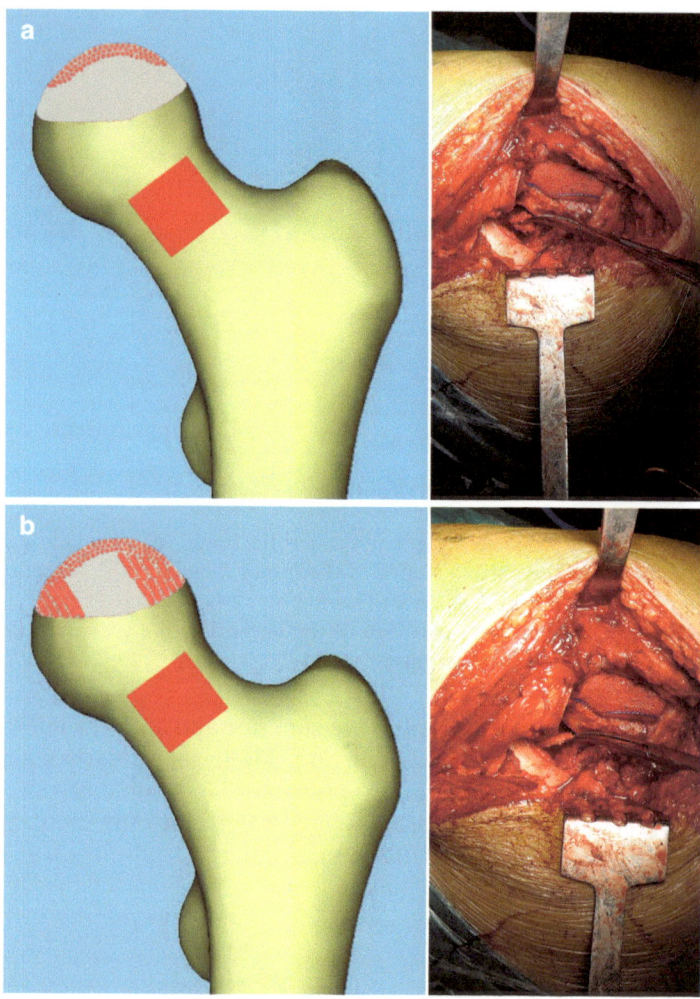

Figure 16.4 Bone grafting. (**a1**, **a2**) The cancellous bone balls and flakes are put onto the inner surface of cartilage of the cavity. (**b1**, **b2**) The many cancellous bone flakes and matchsticks cortical bone strips were planted on inner walls of the empty cavity in the femoral head and pressed solid. A big and long straight passage in the center of the femoral head is reserved, which connected with the fenestration of femoral neck. (**c1**–**c3**) Trim the size of the graft bone pedicled with femoral quadratus

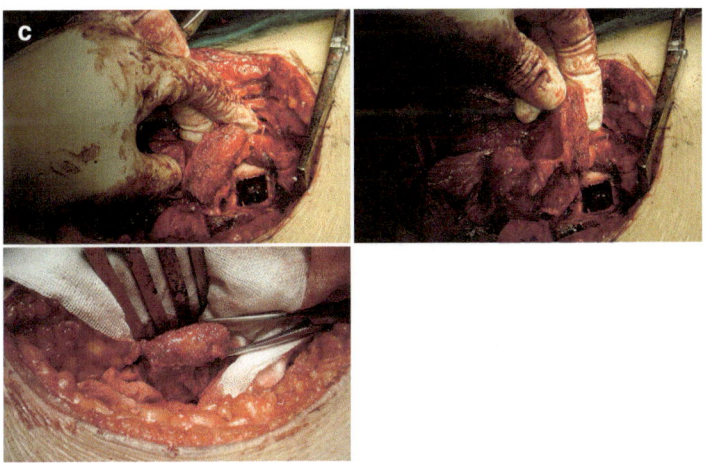

FIGURE 16.4 (continued)

inner walls of the empty cavity in the femoral head and pressed solidly against the walls (Fig. 16.4b1, b2). At the same time, a big and long straight passage in the center of the femoral head is reserved that connects with a fenestration in the femoral neck. The passage will be used for inserting the grafting bone column pedicled with femoral quadratus.

The rectangular bone block needs to be trimmed to become a column of bone that is pedicled with femoral quadratus. Its shape needs to fit a straight passage; its size is usually about $1.4 \times 1.0 \times 4.5$ cm and should be large enough to not damage the vessels of the bone graft (Fig. 16.4c1–c3).

The grafting strut bone column pedicled with femoral quadratus is inserted into the straight passage in the center of the femoral head (Fig. 16.5a, b). The bone column is impacted gently with a metal rod and mallet (Fig. 16.5c), until it completely enters the passage and fenestration groove (Fig. 16.5d). The bone column can support the subchondral bone region and prop up the dome of femoral head proximally and insert into the fenestration groove at the distal side (Fig. 16.5e).

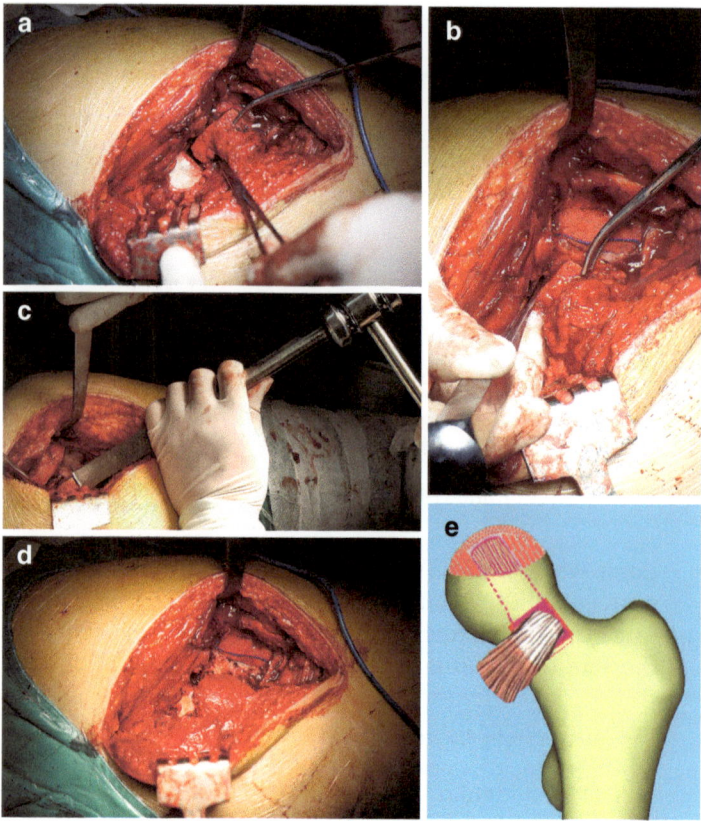

FIGURE 16.5 The strut bone column grafting. (**a–e**) The graft strut bone column pedicle with femoral quadratus is inserted into the straight passage in the center of the femoral head

5. Postoperative treatment:

The patient was restricted to bed rest for the first 3 weeks after surgery, and then the patient was allowed to sit up in bed but not allowed to get up. Partial weight bearing using crutches was allowed at 3 months after the operation when the bone union within the femoral head was seen on radiographs. Full weight bearing was allowed at 5 months after operation.

Outcome

This 31-year-old male patient with preoperative hip pain, limited mobility of the hip, and slight limp presented in this case recovered uneventfully and was able to maintain full mobility of the hip as well as walking normally. The postoperative X-ray films showed thoroughly removed necrotic bone, sufficient grafting bone, and a well-placed strut bone grafting column in the femoral head. X-ray films showed good bone union of the grafting bone and no collapse of the femoral head at 2.3 years after the operation (Fig. 16.6).

Literature Review

For many years, a variety of bone grafting procedures have been used to treat the osteonecrosis of the femoral head (ONFH) in differing necrotic stages. Bone grafting procedures can be vascularized or non-vascularized [1–8]. Vascularized bone graft can restore the blood supply to the femoral head and contribute to its incorporation because of its rich blood supply and ample osteogenic factors. Furthermore, vascularized bone graft can enhance the biomechanical strength of femoral head locally and prevent collapse of the femoral head. This is important, especially for the young patient with a longer life expectancy of the femoral head [3, 9]. Two large categories of vascularized bone grafting are currently used clinically: a free vascularized fibular graft [4, 7, 8] and bone graft pedicled with muscle or some other vascular supply [1, 3, 9–11]. Bone grafting pedicled with femoral quadratus has several important advantages and includes the ability of obtaining the bone block easily, and the operation is relatively simple and practical. Furthermore, the graft bone pedicled with femoral quadratus has a musculoskeletal structure that is directly attached to the graft that has a rich blood supply and a bigger and longer bone column with at least two sides cortical bone can be obtained, so it may be

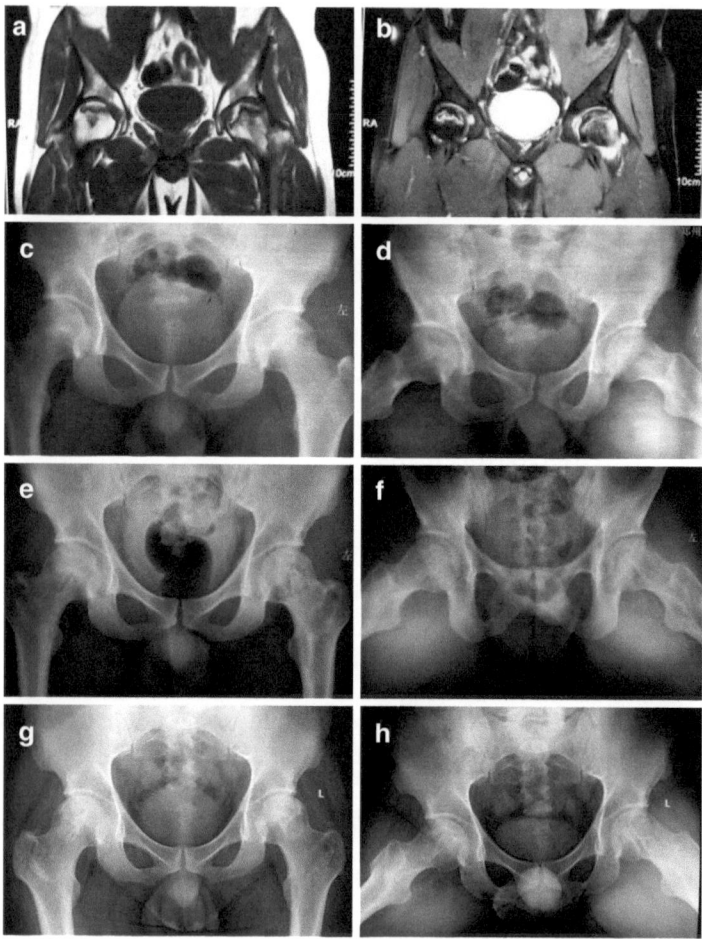

FIGURE 16.6 The bone grafting pedicled with femoral quadratus. A 31-year-old male patient suffered from bilateral alcohol-induced ONFH, *right side* femoral head was in stage ARCO II-B, *left side* was in stage II-C. (**a, b**) Preoperative MRI of bilateral hips. (**c, d**) Preoperative AP and frog-bit X-ray films in *both sides* of femoral heads; (**e, f**) at 1 month postoperative, AP and frog-leg X-ray films, showing thoroughly removed necrotic bone, sufficient grafting bone, and well strut position of grafting bone column in the femoral head. (**g, h**) At 2.3 years postoperative, AP and frog X-ray films, showing good bone union of the grafting bone and no collapse of the femoral head

better for treating pre-collapse ONFH [3, 9, 10]. According to the treatment principles of the Association Research Circulation Osseous (ARCO) classification, the bone grafting is suitable for ONFH in stage II-B, II-C, III-A, and III-B [12]. We have used this technique for ONFH in stage III-A, but the results were not as good as for pre-collapse stages [3]. Eighty two patients with 94 hips with ONFH had surgery with implantation of a quadratus pedicled bone graft and were followed up at least 3 years. Thirty six, 30, and 28 hips were in the stage ARCO II-B, II-C, and III-A, respectively. Pain in the hip area in all patients disappeared or mostly relieved after surgery. Hip range of motion improved. The follow-up time was from 0.5 to 5.5 years with an average of 3.2 years. The rate of excellent and good results was 94.4%, 93.3%, and 89.3% in stage II-B, II-C, and III-A, respectively. The rate of excellent and good in total was 92.6%. The outcome in this group proved that the bone grafting pedicled with femoral quadratus is especially applicable for ONFH in stage II-B and II-C in younger patients [3].

Clinical Pearls and Pitfalls

- The necrotic area is usually located in the superior and anterior-lateral region in the femoral head and can be seen clearly during this procedure performed through the posterior approach. The necrotic bone must be completely removed.
- Take care and do not cut through or scratch and perforate the cartilage layer.
- The grafting strut bone column pedicled with femoral quadratus can support subchondral bone region and prop up the dome of femoral head proximally and, when inserted into the fenestration groove at the distal side, improve the biomechanical properties of femoral head and can repair and prevent collapse of the femoral head.

- How to avoid fracture of the bone strut:

  1. Do not take rude chisel.
  2. Trim the rectangular bone block so that it becomes a grafting strut of bone column pedicled on the femoral quadratus and its size fits to insert smoothly into the straight passage, so that it does not get stuck or fracture in the implanting process.
  3. The bone column is impacted gently with a metal rod and hammer, until it completely enters the passage and fenestration groove.

- How to mobilize the quadratus: The bone column is rotated around 90 degree to enter the passage within the femoral head. The femoral quadratus, muscle pedicle of the bone column, is loose and long enough. It can be moved easily without difficulty.
- How to know where to split the quadratus: Must carefully separate the upper and lower edges of the femoral quadratus. After the rectangular bone block is taken with chisel, the femoral quadratus should be peeled from its deep surface. Its blood supply should be protected.
- How do we start bony harvest: After the complete removal of necrotic bone, there will be a large cavity that will require bone grafting. Plan to obtain sufficient bone for grafting: (1) matchstick-shaped cortical bone strips, (2) cancellous bone pellets and flakes, and (3) a larger strut bone column pedicled with femoral quadratus.
- How to avoid the damage to the blood supply: (1) Carefully cut off the muscle attachment points of the obturator and gemelli on the femur. (2) Don't damage the attachment part on the bone column of femoral quadratus muscle pedicle to avoid damaging the blood supply when trimming the rectangular bone block to become a column of bone.

- Limit range of motion of the hip: The patient is restricted to bed rest for the first 3 weeks after operation, legs at abduction position around 30°~45°, and then patient can sit up and move on bed, but can't get up and weight bearing. Partial weight bearing using crutches is allowed at 3 months or longer after the operation when the bone union within the femoral head is seen on the X-ray film. Full weight bearing is allowed at 2 months after partial weight bearing using crutches when the femoral head is no collapse in the X-ray films.

Acknowledgments The author thanks his PhD candidate Shang Guowei, M.D. (Zhengzhou University, Zhengzhou, Henan, China), for helping with the preparation of this chapter.

References

1. Meyers MH. Osteonecrosis of the femoral head treated with the muscle pedicle graft. Orthop CIin North Am. 1985;16(4):741–5.
2. Vahid Farahmandi M, Abbasian M, Safdari F, Emami Moghaddam Tehrani M. Midterm results of treating femoral head osteonecrosis with autogenous cortico cancellous bone grafting. Trauma Mon. 2014;19(4):e17092.
3. Wang YS, Yin L, Wu XJ, Liu HJ. Bone grafting pedicled with muscle for osteonecrosis of femoral head. Chin J Joint Surg. 2008;2(1):3–6.
4. Kim SY, Kim YG, Kim PT, Ihn JC, Cho BC, Koo KH. Vascularized compared with nonvascularized fibular grafts for large osteonecrotic lesions of the femoral head. J Bone Joint Surg Am. 2005;87(9):2012–8.
5. Meyers MH. The treatment of osteonecrosis of the hip with fresh osteochondral allografts and with the muscle pedicle graft technique. Clin Orthop Relat Res. 1978;130:202–9.
6. Mont MA, Jones LC, Hungerford DS. Nontraumatic osteonecrosis of the femoral head: ten years later. J Bone Joint Surg Am. 2006;88(5):1117–32.

7. Aldridge 3rd JM, Urbaniak JR. Avascular necrosis of the femoral head: role of vascularized bone grafts. Orthop Clin North Am. 2007;38(1):13–22.

8. Korompilias AV, Beris AE, Lykissas MG, Kostas-Agnantis IP, Soucacos PN. Femoral head osteonecrosis: why choose free vascularized fibula grafting. Microsurgery. 2011;31(3):223–8.

9. Wang YS, Zhang Y, Li JW, Yang GH, Li JF, Yang J, Yang GH. A modified technique of bone grafting pedicled with femoral quadratus for alcohol-induced osteonecrosis of the femoral head. Chin Med J (Engl). 2010;123(20):2847–52.

10. Wang YS, Yin L, Lu ZD, Wu XJ, Liu HJ. Analysis of long-term outcomes of double-strut bone graft for osteonecrosis of the femoral head. Ortho Surg. 2009;1(1):22–7.

11. Zhao D, Yu X, Wang T, Wang B, Liu B, Tian F, Fu W, Huang S, Qiu X. Digital subtraction angiography in selection of the vascularized greater trochanter bone grafting for treatment ofosteonecrosis of femoral head. Microsurgery. 2013;33(8):656–9.

12. Cui Q, Wang Y, Wang G-J. Femoral head necrosis. In: Luo X, Qiu G, editors. Surgery of artificial hip replacement. 1st ed. Peking: Peking Union Medical College Publication; 2003. p. 275–9.

Chapter 17

Transtrochanteric Anterior Rotational Osteotomy of the Femoral Head for Treatment of Osteonecrosis Affecting the Hip

Cody C. Wyles, Rafael J. Sierra, and Robert T. Trousdale

Case Presentation

A 37-year-old gentleman presented with progressive right groin pain of 1-year duration. He had no prior history of trauma or previous difficulty with his hips. His problem began as thigh pain after extended walks and progressed to deep groin pain with prolonged standing or tying his shoes. The discomfort was intermittently

C.C. Wyles, BS • R.J. Sierra, MD • R.T. Trousdale, MD (✉)
Department of Orthopaedic Surgery, Mayo Clinic,
Rochester, MN 55905, USA
e-mail: trousdale.robert@mayo.edu

R.J. Sierra (ed.), *Osteonecrosis of the Femoral Head*,
DOI 10.1007/978-3-319-50664-7_17,
© Mayo Foundation for Medical Education and Research 2017

189

present at night and became severe enough with activity to limit his ability to work. He had no identifiable risk factors for ON of the femoral head other than occasional use of alcohol.

On physical examination, the patient was a tall, thin Caucasian male. He walked with a non-antalgic, even gait and did not exhibit a Trendelenburg sign. Range of motion of the left hip was full and painless, whereas on the right his passive range of motion was marked by full extension, 115° flexion, 35° external rotation, 0° internal rotation, 50° abduction, and 30° adduction. His leg lengths were equal and he achieved adequate toe and heel walking. Strength, sensation, and reflexes were shown to be equal and full bilaterally in the lower extremities.

Diagnosis/Assessment

AP radiograph of the pelvis demonstrated slight irregularity and sclerosis of the right femoral head consistent with ON (Fig. 17.1a). Bone scan of the pelvis documented increased uptake in the right proximal femur (Fig. 17.1b) surrounding a central core with decreased uptake on the pinhole view (not available), also consistent with ON. He was initially made to do toe-touch weight-bearing on crutches for 2 months; nevertheless, his symptoms were unabated by this conservative approach. Given the patient's progressive pain, physical examination, and imaging findings, the decision was made to pursue operative intervention. He presented only a few years after the first description of Sugioka osteotomy; however, a surgeon at our institution had already begun to use the technique as a joint preservation strategy for patients with early stage ON of the femoral head. He was counseled on the risks and benefits inherent to both Sugioka osteotomy and THA in

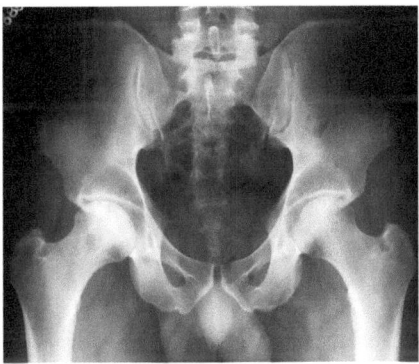 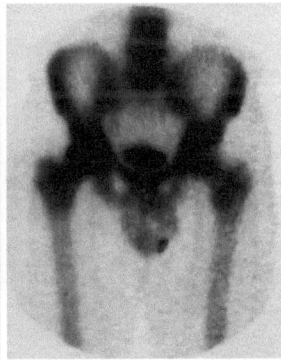

FIGURE 17.1 AP radiograph of the pelvis demonstrates slight irregularity and sclerosis of the right femoral head consistent with ON (**a**). Bone scan of the pelvis documents increased uptake in the right proximal femur (**b**). The pinhole view of this bone scan was unavailable; however, the radiologist report describes a central core with decreased uptake, also consistent with ON

the early 1980s and subsequently elected to undergo transtrochanteric anterior rotational osteotomy.

Management

The patient was treated with a transtrochanteric anterior rotational osteotomy as follows. In the lateral decubitus position, the hip was exposed through a lateral approach. The external rotators were detached from the posterior greater trochanter taking care to respect the quadratus femoris and the medial circumflex femoral artery. The trochanter was osteotomized and retracted proximally, holding it to the ilium with a Charnley spike. A capsulotomy was performed at the level of the labrum and carried out circumferentially both anteriorly and posteriorly, as well as medially. Two guide wires were driven across the cut surface of the greater trochanter aiming them at the lesser trochanter so that they were parallel to each other, one anterior and one posterior and both perpendicular to the longitudinal axis of the femur. The position of the guide wires was proven by X-ray, and then a primary osteotomy was made along the plane provided by the two guide wires. A secondary osteotomy was then created perpendicular to the first. The proximal fragment was subsequently rotated anteriorly utilizing two heavy pins, one placed in the proximal fragment and one in the distal fragment to effect this rotation. The osteotomy was held together with a Lane clamp, and a guide wire was driven across the osteotomy along with two 3.2 mm antirotation drills. The position of the guide wire and drills was proven by X-ray, and a super lag screw was placed in the femoral head. The vastus lateralis was elevated from the femur at the level of the intermuscular septum, and a 130° long-barrel side plate was incorporated into the super lag screw and fixed to the femur with four non-self-tapping screws. One of the 3.2 mm drills was removed and replaced with a 65 mm long threaded antirotational cancellous screw. The capsule was closed with 0 Vicryl sutures and the greater trochanter reattached with two crossed #18 stainless steel wire sutures. The vastus lateralis was reattached over the plate with 0 Vicryl and the external rotators attached to the greater trochanter. Additional closure was performed in a standard fashion.

Following the procedure, he was kept to toe-touch weight-bearing on crutches for 3 months and then allowed to slowly advance his weight-bearing as tolerated. He was completely asymptomatic by 1 year with resolution of his postoperative limp.

Outcome

This 37-year-old man with ON of the femoral head was initially treated with a transtrochanteric anterior rotational osteotomy (Fig. 17.2). Pain and functionality were improved for 3 years after the procedure. The distal tip of the Richards screw in his operative construct had an asymptomatic break, which was documented at the 6-month follow-up visit (Fig. 17.3). Eventually, his disease progressed and collapse of the femoral head with increased pain was documented at

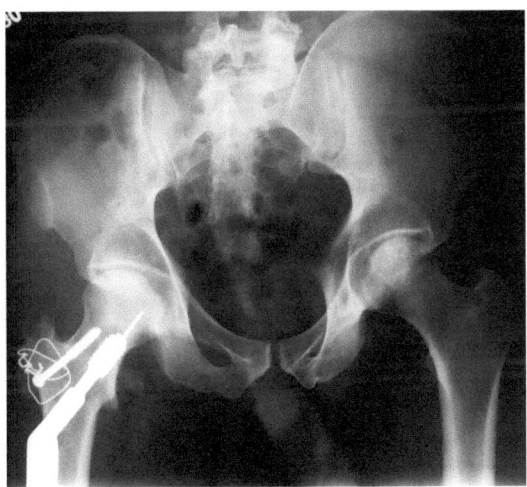

FIGURE 17.2 AP radiograph of the pelvis 3 months status post-transtrochanteric anterior rotational osteotomy demonstrates the osteotomized proximal femur with a spherical portion of the femoral head occupying the weight-bearing zone

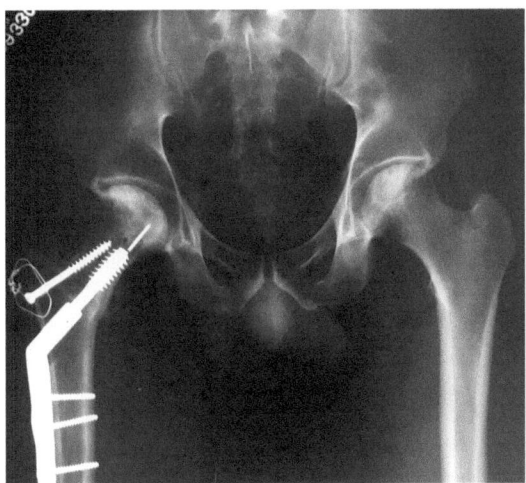

FIGURE 17.3 AP radiograph of the pelvis 6 months status post-transtrochanteric anterior rotational osteotomy demonstrates fracture of the distal tip of the Richards screw. This was asymptomatic and the construct was otherwise stable

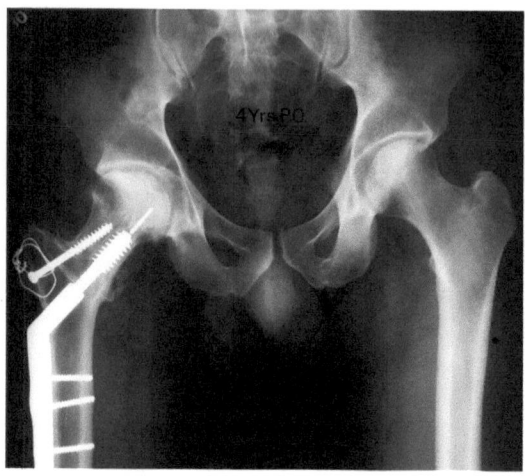

FIGURE 17.4 AP radiograph of the pelvis 4 years status post-transtrochanteric anterior rotational osteotomy demonstrates increased irregularity of the femoral head with sclerosis, cyst formation, and collapse. This radiograph correlated with pain during any weight-bearing activities

4-year follow-up (Fig. 17.4). At this point, it was determined that THA provided the most reliable option to manage his condition. He received an uncemented THA (Fig. 17.5), which resolved his pain and allowed full-time return to work. The prosthesis has remained without complication for 23 years; however, mild superior migration of the femoral head from polyethylene wear and what appears to be significant osteolysis of the superior aspect of the acetabulum are noted radiographically (Fig. 17.6).

Literature Review

There are few large reports concerning transtrochanteric anterior rotational osteotomy, particularly in the recent peer-reviewed literature as use of the procedure is now largely

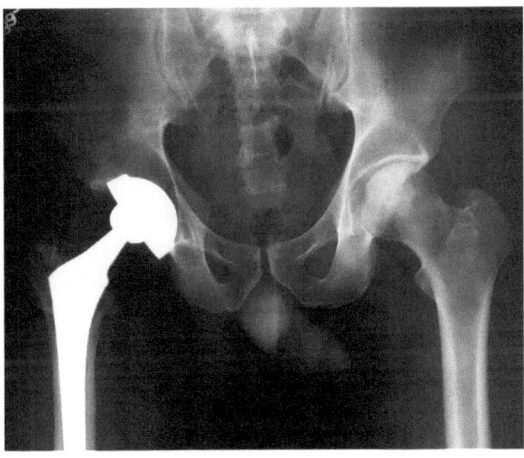

FIGURE 17.5 AP radiograph of the pelvis 3 months status post-uncemented THA with well-fixed and well-positioned components

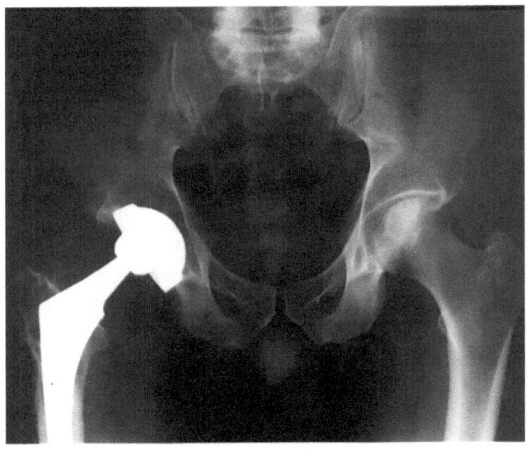

FIGURE 17.6 AP radiograph of the pelvis 23 years status post-uncemented THA demonstrates mild proximal migration of the femoral head component secondary to polyethylene wear. Supra-acetabular osteolysis is noted; however, the construct is otherwise functionally stable

restricted to Japan. When Sugioka first published a description of the technique in 1978, he reported outcomes on 41 hips out of the first 80 to receive the operation for ON of the femoral head [1]. At mean follow-up of 2.5 years, 85% remained free from femoral head collapse, 88% had no recurrence of pain, and 90% had no reduction in their range of motion. A subsequent report by Sugioka in 1992 documented a success rate of 78% in 295 hips over 3–16-year follow-up [2]. No other reports in the peer-reviewed literature to date have rivaled the success reported by Sugioka and colleagues.

By contrast to results from Japan, a single surgeon experience from our institution described outcomes in 18 hips with ON of the femoral head managed by transtrochanteric anterior rotational osteotomy [3]. Mean follow-up in this cohort was 57 months (range 18–106). Among the 18 hips under study, 15 (83%) were determined to have a clinically poor outcome as defined by progression to THA within the study period. One notable difference in the postoperative protocol for this cohort was advancement to weight-bearing as tolerated following radiographic documentation of osteotomy union. The mean time to union for the cohort was 10 weeks – the patient described in the case report above achieved radiographic union at 12 weeks. Sugioka and colleagues have advocated for 6 months non-weight-bearing following transtrochanteric anterior rotational osteotomy.

Another report by Rijnen et al. details outcomes from their center following transtrochanteric anterior rotational osteotomy performed by a surgeon who learned the technique directly from Sugioka in Japan [4]. They report that after a mean follow-up of 4.7 years (range 1.4–10.1), 17 of 26 hips (65%) were converted to THA despite strictly adhering to the postoperative protocol suggested by Sugioka. These authors subsequently described the additional challenges posed during THA following a previous transtrochanteric anterior rotational osteotomy. The comparison group was 17 hips that received THA after failure of bone impaction grafting as initial joint preservation therapy for ON of the femoral head. In the osteotomy group, they describe anatomical distortion, unrecognizable external rotators, and fibrous tissue formation as ubiquitous challenges. Furthermore, they state that locating/removing screws and cerclage wires could not be adequately performed in four cases and that preoperative templating was inaccurate in nearly every case. By contrast, no perioperative complications were observed in the bone impaction grafting group. In additional comparisons between patients with previous osteotomy versus bone impaction grafting, they report statistically significant differences in THA outcomes including postoperative complications (radiologic loosening, infection, and dislocations), as well as operative time, perioperative blood loss, and length of hospital stay, with all outcomes being worse in the osteotomy group. In summary, not only was the transtrochanteric anterior rotational osteotomy a poor temporizing measure for joint preservation, but it also led to significantly worse outcomes with subsequent THA.

Clinical Pearls and Pitfalls

- Transtrochanteric anterior rotational osteotomy as described by Sugioka is a technically demanding procedure. The excellent results achieved in Japan by Sugioka and colleagues have not been replicated by other surgeons.
- The success of this operation rests on the ability to carefully maintain the blood supply to the femoral head. In particular the medial circumflex femoral artery and retinacular arteries must not be violated.
- THA following failed Sugioka osteotomy can pose unique technical challenges, with significantly higher perioperative and postoperative complication rates. As other joint preservation techniques have matured in parallel with the expanding indications for THA, Sugioka osteotomy should be reserved for very select cases in only the most experienced hands.

References

1. Sugioka Y. Transtrochanteric anterior rotational osteotomy of the femoral head in the treatment of osteonecrosis affecting the hip: a new osteotomy operation. Clin Orthop Relat Res. 1978;130:191–201.
2. Sugioka Y, Hotokebuchi T, Tsutsui H. Transtrochanteric anterior rotational osteotomy for idiopathic and steroid-induced necrosis of the femoral head. Indications and long-term results. Clin Orthopaed Rel Res. 1992;277:111–20.
3. Dean MT, Cabanela ME. Transtrochanteric anterior rotational osteotomy for avascular necrosis of the femoral head. Long-term results. J Bone Joint Surg Br Volume. 1993;75(4):597–601.
4. Rijnen WH, et al. Total hip arthroplasty after failed treatment for osteonecrosis of the femoral head. Orthopedic Clin N Am. 2009;40(2):291–8.

Part III
Post-collapse: Arthroplasty and Complications

Chapter 18
Systemic Lupus Erythematosus Patient Requiring THA

Todd P. Pierce, Julio J. Jauregui, Jeffrey J. Cherian, Randa K. Elmallah, and Michael A. Mont

Case Presentation

A 64-year-old woman presented with a 1-year history of spontaneous onset right hip pain. She has a history of systemic lupus erythematosis and myositis, previously treated with high-dose corticosteroids. She had been experiencing mild pain on walking, going up and down-stairs, and at rest. She had also developed a moderate limp but denied use of walking aids. On presentation to clinic, she was still taking prednisone 2.5 milligrams daily. The patient had been told at an outside hospital that she would benefit from core decompression. Other past medical history was significant for hypertension and anemia.

T.P. Pierce, MD • J.J. Jauregui, MD • J.J. Cherian, DO
R.K. Elmallah, MD • M.A. Mont, MD (✉)
Center for Joint Preservation and Replacement, Rubin Institute for Advanced Orthopaedics, Sinai Hospital of Baltimore,
2401 West Belvedere Avenue, Baltimore, MD 21215, USA
e-mail: tpierce@gwmail.gwu.edu; juljau@gmail.com;
jjaicherian@gmail.com; randaelmallah@gmail.com;
mmont@lifebridgehealth.org; rhondamont@aol.com

R.J. Sierra (ed.), *Osteonecrosis of the Femoral Head*,
DOI 10.1007/978-3-319-50664-7_18,
© Mayo Foundation for Medical Education and Research 2017

201

Diagnosis/Assessment

Initial x-rays showed post-collapse disease with acetabular involvement in the right hip (See Fig. 18.1).

Management

After consultation, the patient was informed of the post-collapse disease within the right hip. At that point, she was counseled that core decompression would not benefit her, and she agreed to proceed with a total hip arthroplasty. Informed consent was obtained after discussing the risks and benefits of the planned procedures prior to surgery.

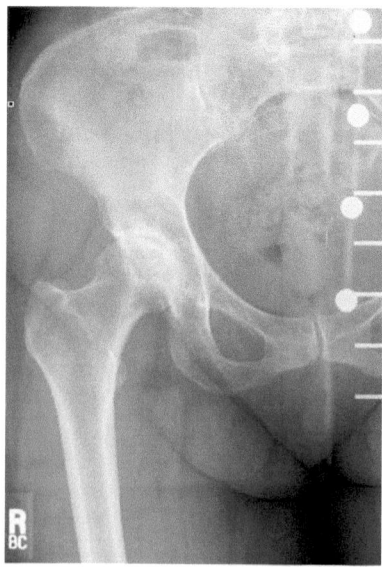

FIGURE 18.1 Preoperative radiographs showing femoral head collapse and acetabular involvement

Total Hip Arthroplasty

The patient was placed in the left lateral decubitus position. We prepped and draped the right hip in the usual aseptic manner. A time-out was performed prior to the incision. A 14-cm skin incision was made over the greater trochanter for an anterolateral approach to the hip and deepened down through the skin and subcutaneous tissue through the fascia lata. We took off the anterior 40% of the gluteus medius, removed the minimus, and performed a capsulectomy. We then dislocated the femoral head and removed it. At that time, we noted significant degenerative disease in the femoral head. We reamed the acetabulum and placed it in a press-fit construct. We took off the peripheral osteophytes and put in a neutral polyethylene liner. We then prepared the stem with the appropriate-sized stem and head combination. We achieved excellent stability and excellent leg length.

After careful irrigation, closure of the muscles, subcutaneous tissue, and skin was performed, and a sterile dressing was applied. The patient was then taken to the recovery room in stable condition.

Outcome

At her 3-month follow-up, she was pain-free and performing all her daily activities without difficulty. Radiographic evaluation showed a well-placed arthroplasty without evidence of osteolysis or loosening (See Fig. 18.2). On physical exam, the patient had minimal peri-incisional tenderness. She had five out of five muscular strengths and was neurovascularly intact at the lower extremities.

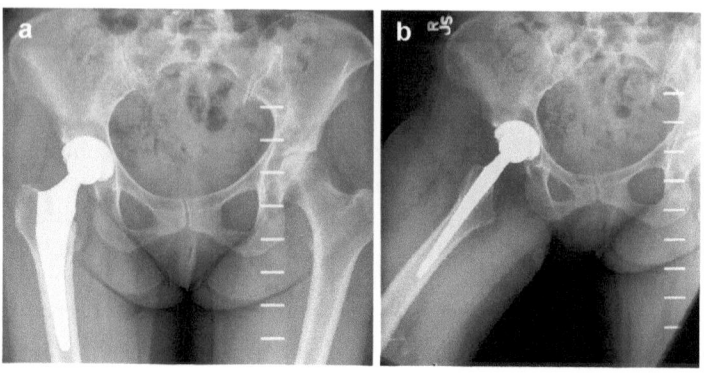

FIGURE 18.2 (**a**, **b**) Post-THA radiographs showing a well-placed implant with no signs of loosening or fracture

Clinical Pearls and Pitfalls

- SLE patients may have damage to the articular cartilage that was not noted in preoperative imaging, so it is critical to have the equipment needed to convert to THA if you are attempting any hip-preserving procedures.

Literature Review

Patients with SLE can derive great benefit from THA. However, there are five small studies with midterm follow-up outcomes with two of these studies being comparative. Future studies should have larger cohorts with long-term follow-up (See Table 18.1).

TABLE 18.1 Outcomes of THA in ON patients with osteonecrosis

Author, year	Case cohort description	Number of cases	Number of controls	Mean follow-up, months (range)	Cases' mean HHS, points	Controls' mean HHS, points	Cases' implant survivorship, %	Controls' implant survivorship, %
Graham et al. (2014) [1]	HIV	43	–	42 (5–98)	86	–	100	–
Issa et al. (2013) [2]	HIV	44	78	84 (48–132)	85	87	95	96.5
Issa et al. (2013) [3]	SLE	60	82	84 (48–132)	87	88	98	97.5
Kim et al. (2013) [4]	Age < 50 years	64	–	189 (180–201)	93	–	93.8	–
Kang et al. (2013) [5]	SLE	28	–	68 (12–156)	84	–	100	–
Chang et al. (2013) [6]	Post-kidney transplant	74	–	122 (60–197)	89	–	97	–

(continued)

Table 18.1 (continued)

Author, year	Case cohort description	Number of cases	Number of controls	Mean follow-up, months (range)	Cases' mean HHS, points	Controls' mean HHS, points	Cases' implant survivorship, %	Controls' implant survivorship, %
Wang et al. (2013) [7]	Age > 80 years	92	–	72 (60–144)	80	–	95	–
Han et al. (2013) [8]	All ON etiologies	95	–	152 (128–207)	92	–	98.9	–
Zangger et al. (2000) [9]	SLE	26	29	55 (21–114)	87	82	96	100
Chen et al. (1999) [10]	SLE	18	–	45 (24–85)	96	–	100	–
Huo et al. (1992) [11]	SLE	33	–	52 (24–108)	–	–	94.6	–

References

1. Graham SM, Lubega N, Mkandawire N, Harrison WJ. Total hip replacement in HIV-positive patients. Bone Joint J. 2014;96-B(4):462–6.
2. Issa K, Naziri Q, Rasquinha V, Maheshwari AV, Delanois RE, Mont MA. Outcomes of cementless primary THA for osteonecrosis in HIV-infected patients. J Bone Joint Surg Am. 2013;95(20):1845–50.
3. Issa K, Naziri Q, Rasquinha VJ, Tatevossian T, Kapadia BH, Mont MA. Outcomes of primary total hip arthroplasty in systemic lupus erythematosus with a proximally-coated cementless stem. J Arthroplast. 2013;28(9):1663–6.
4. Kim SM, Lim SJ, Moon YW, Kim YT, Ko KR, Park YS. Cementless modular total hip arthroplasty in patients younger than fifty with femoral head osteonecrosis: minimum fifteen-year follow-up. J Arthroplast. 2013;28(3):504–9.
5. Kang Y, Zhang ZJ, Zhao XY, Zhang ZQ, Sheng PY, Liao WM. Total hip arthroplasty for vascular necrosis of the femoral head in patients with systemic lupus erythematosus: a midterm follow-up study of 28 hips in 24 patients. Eur J Orthopaedic Surg Traumatol Orthopedie Traumatol. 2013;23(1):73–9.
6. Chang JS, Han DJ, Park SK, Sung JH, Ha YC. Cementless total hip arthroplasty in patients with osteonecrosis after kidney transplantation. J Arthroplast. 2013;28(5):824–7.
7. Wang TI, Hung SH, Su YP, Feng CQ, Chiu FY, Liu CL. Noncemented total hip arthroplasty for osteonecrosis of the femoral head in elderly patients. Orthopedics. 2013;36(3):e271–5.
8. Han SI, Lee JH, Kim JW, Oh CW, Kim SY. Long-term durability of the CLS femoral prosthesis in patients with osteonecrosis of the femoral head. J Arthroplast. 2013;28(5):828–31.
9. Zangger P, Gladman DD, Urowitz MB, Bogoch ER. Outcome of total hip replacement for avascular necrosis in systemic lupus erythematosus. J Rheumatol. 2000;27(4):919–23.
10. Chen YW, Chang JK, Huang KY, Lin GT, Lin SY, Huang CY. Hip arthroplasty for osteonecrosis in patients with systemic lupus erythematosus. Kaohsiung J Med Sci. 1999;15(12):697–703.
11. Huo MH, Salvati EA, Browne MG, Pellicci PM, Sculco TP, Johanson NA. Primary total hip arthroplasty in systemic lupus erythematosus. J Arthroplast. 1992;7(1):51–6.

Chapter 19
Attempted Bone Grafting Converted Intraoperatively to THA

Todd P. Pierce, Julio J. Jauregui, Jeffrey J. Cherian, Randa K. Elmallah, and Michael A. Mont

Case Presentation

A 50-year-old woman presented with an 18-month history of right hip pain. She complained of moderate pain when walking and going up and downstairs with mild pain at rest. Other past medical history was significant for hypertension and anemia.

T.P. Pierce, MD • J.J. Jauregui, MD • J.J. Cherian, DO
R.K. Elmallah, MD • M.A. Mont, MD (✉)
Center for Joint Preservation and Replacement, Rubin Institute for Advanced Orthopaedics, Sinai Hospital of Baltimore, 2401 West Belvedere Avenue, Baltimore, MD 21215, USA
e-mail: tpierce@gwmail.gwu.edu; juljau@gmail.com; jjaicherian@gmail.com; randaelmallah@gmail.com; mmont@lifebridgehealth.org; rhondamont@aol.com

R.J. Sierra (ed.), *Osteonecrosis of the Femoral Head*,
DOI 10.1007/978-3-319-50664-7_19,
© Mayo Foundation for Medical Education and Research 2017

Diagnosis/Assessment

Initial radiographs approximately 2 weeks prior to surgery showed Ficat stage II ON of the right hip (see Fig. 19.1).

Management

After consultation, the patient was counseled that it would be best to proceed with a nonvascularized bone grafting as he preferred to delay THA by all means possible. Informed consent was obtained after discussing the risks and benefits of the planned procedures prior to surgery, including the risk of converting to a THA. Although the patient was aware that we would proceed bone grafting, she communicated that we may have to convert to a THA if we saw damage to the articular cartilage or signs of collapse not otherwise seen.

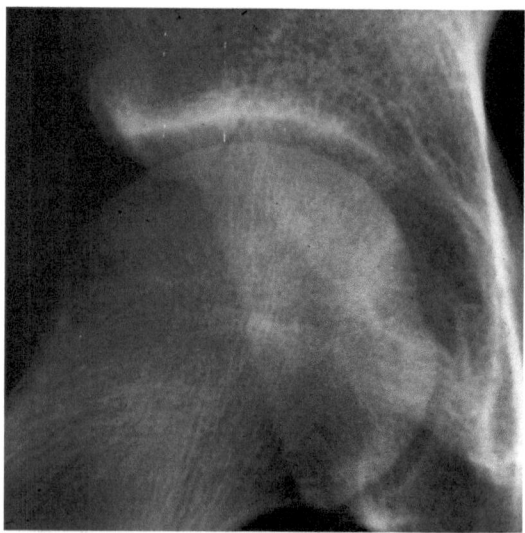

FIGURE 19.1 Preoperative radiographs showing no acetabular involvement

Bone Grafting

A 15-cm incision was made through an anterolateral approach, deepened it down through the skin and subcutaneous tissue and through the fascia lata. We took off the anterior 40% of the gluteus medius and minimus. We did a capsulectomy. When exposing the hip joint, we noticed there was significant degeneration of the femoral head with damage to the articular cartilage (see Fig. 19.2). At this time, we deemed grafting to be an insufficient treatment and elected to convert to a total hip replacement.

Total Hip Arthroplasty

We reamed the acetabulum and placed it in a press-fit construct. We took off the peripheral osteophytes and put in a neutral polyethylene liner. We then prepared the stem with

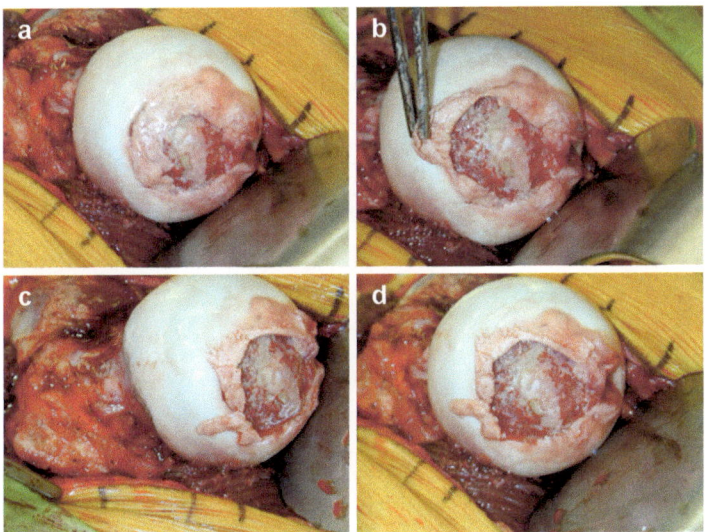

FIGURE 19.2 (**a–d**) Intraoperative examination of the right hip showing damage to the intra-articular cartilage

the appropriate-sized stem and head combination. We achieved excellent stability and excellent leg length.

After careful irrigation, closure of the muscles, subcutaneous tissue, and skin was performed, and a sterile dressing was applied. The patient was then taken to the recovery room in stable condition.

Outcome

At her 14-week follow-up, she was pain-free and performing all her daily activities without difficulty. Radiographic evaluation showed a well-placed arthroplasty without evidence of osteolysis or loosening (See Fig. 19.3). On physical exam, the patient had minimal peri-incisional tenderness. She had five

FIGURE 19.3 Postoperative radiographs showing a well-placed implant with no signs of loosening or fracture

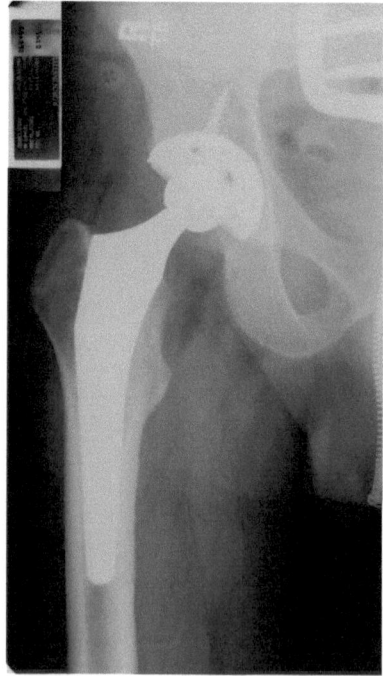

out of five muscular strengths and was neurovascularly intact at the lower extremities. The outcomes of THA in patients with ON are shown in Table 19.1.

Clinical Pearls and Pitfalls

- Damage to articular cartilage may not be seen on imaging studies, so the equipment to convert to THA must be available if intraoperative examination reveals damage.
- Must convert to THA if:
  - Inadequate bone stock in the acetabulum or femoral head and neck based on clinical judgment
  - Degeneration within the articular cartilage

TABLE 19.1 Outcomes of THA in patients with osteonecrosis

Author, year	Case cohort	Cement vs. cementless	Number of cases	Number of controls	Mean follow-up, months (range)	Case mean HHS, points	Control mean HHS, points	Case implant survivorship, %	Control implant survivorship, %
Graham et al. (2014) [1]	HIV	Cement	43	–	42 (5–98)	86	–	100	–
Issa et al. (2013) [2]	HIV	Cementless	44	78	84 (48–132)	85	87	95	96.5
Issa et al. (2013) [3]	SLE	Cementless	60	82	84 (48–132)	87	88	98	97.5
Kim et al. (2013) [4]	Age < 50 years	Cementless	64	–	189 (180–201)	93	–	93.8	–
Kang et al. (2013) [5]	SLE	Cementless femur; majority cementless acetabulum (24)	28	–	68 (12–156)	84	–	100	–

Chang et al. (2013) [6]	Post-kidney transplant	Cementless	74	–	122 (60–197)	89	–	97	–
Wang et al. (2013) [7]	Age > 80 years	Cementless	92	–	72 (60–144)	80	–	95	–
Han et al. (2013) [8]	All ON etiologies	Cementless	95	–	152 (128–207)	92	–	98.9	–
Zangger et al. (2000) [9]	SLE	–	26	29	55 (21–114)	87	82	96	100
Chen et al. (1999) [10]	SLE	–	18	–	45 (24–85)	96	–	100	–
Huo et al. (1992) [11]	SLE	Cemented	33	–	52 (24–108)	–	–	94.6	–

References

1. Graham SM, Lubega N, Mkandawire N, Harrison WJ. Total hip replacement in HIV-positive patients. Bone Joint J. 2014;96-B(4):462–6.
2. Issa K, Naziri Q, Rasquinha V, Maheshwari AV, Delanois RE, Mont MA. Outcomes of cementless primary THA for osteonecrosis in HIV-infected patients. J Bone Joint Surg Am. 2013;95(20):1845–50.
3. Issa K, Naziri Q, Rasquinha VJ, Tatevossian T, Kapadia BH, Mont MA. Outcomes of primary total hip arthroplasty in systemic lupus erythematosus with a proximally-coated cementless stem. J Arthroplast. 2013;28(9):1663–6.
4. Kim SM, Lim SJ, Moon YW, Kim YT, Ko KR, Park YS. Cementless modular total hip arthroplasty in patients younger than fifty with femoral head osteonecrosis: minimum fifteen-year follow-up. J Arthroplast. 2013;28(3):504–9.
5. Kang Y, Zhang ZJ, Zhao XY, Zhang ZQ, Sheng PY, Liao WM. Total hip arthroplasty for vascular necrosis of the femoral head in patients with systemic lupus erythematosus: a midterm follow-up study of 28 hips in 24 patients. Eur J Orthopaed Surg Traumatol Orthopedie Traumatol. 2013;23(1):73–9.
6. Chang JS, Han DJ, Park SK, Sung JH, Ha YC. Cementless total hip arthroplasty in patients with osteonecrosis after kidney transplantation. J Arthroplast. 2013;28(5):824–7.
7. Wang TI, Hung SH, Su YP, Feng CQ, Chiu FY, Liu CL. Noncemented total hip arthroplasty for osteonecrosis of the femoral head in elderly patients. Orthopedics. 2013;36(3):e271–5.
8. Han SI, Lee JH, Kim JW, Oh CW, Kim SY. Long-term durability of the CLS femoral prosthesis in patients with osteonecrosis of the femoral head. J Arthroplast. 2013;28(5):828–31.
9. Zangger P, Gladman DD, Urowitz MB, Bogoch ER. Outcome of total hip replacement for avascular necrosis in systemic lupus erythematosus. J Rheumatol. 2000;27(4):919–23.
10. Chen YW, Chang JK, Huang KY, Lin GT, Lin SY, Huang CY. Hip arthroplasty for osteonecrosis in patients with systemic lupus erythematosus. Kaohsiung J Med Sci. 1999;15(12):697–703.
11. Huo MH, Salvati EA, Browne MG, Pellicci PM, Sculco TP, Johanson NA. Primary total hip arthroplasty in systemic lupus erythematosus. J Arthroplast. 1992;7(1):51–6.

Chapter 20
All Osteonecroses Are Not Predictor of Poor Outcome with Cemented Total Hip Arthroplasty: A 30-Year Follow-Up Case Presentation with Bilateral Ceramic on Ceramic Bearing Surface

Philippe Hernigou, Arnaud Dubory, Damien Potage, and Charles Henri Flouzat Lachaniette

Case Presentation

A 29-year-old patient complained in 1983 of bilateral medial thigh and groin pain with limitation of hip motion. Symptoms were amplified with weight bearing and relieved with rest but recently increased in the night and irradiated in knees.

P. Hernigou, MD (✉) • C.H.F. Lachaniette, MD
Professor of Orthopaedic Surgery, University Paris East,
Department of Orthopaedic Surgery, 51 avenue du Maréchal de
Lattre de Tassigny, 94010 cedex, Créteil, France
e-mail: philippe.hernigou@wanadoo.fr

A. Dubory, MD • D. Potage, MD
University Paris East, Department of Orthopaedic Surgery,
51 avenue du Maréchal de Lattre de Tassigny,
94010 cedex, Créteil, France

R.J. Sierra (ed.), *Osteonecrosis of the Femoral Head*,
DOI 10.1007/978-3-319-50664-7_20,
© Mayo Foundation for Medical Education and Research 2017

217

Diagnosis/Assessment

Range of motion becomes limited, particularly hip abduction and internal rotation, and passive internal elicits pain. Radiographs demonstrated bilateral hip osteonecrosis with collapse, advanced disease of the femoral head, and flattening. Osteoarthritic joint space narrowing with osteophyte formation was present in one hip. No specific cause of osteonecrosis was found except increased level of cholesterolemia and triglyceridemia.

Management

The patient received in 1983 bilateral cemented total hip arthroplasty (THA) with ceramic on ceramic bearing.

Outcomes

Thirty-three years later in 2016, the patient is hip pain-free, but presents cardiac disease in relation with hypercholesterolemia and hypertriglyceridemia.

Literature Review

Disease Presentation

The association between lipid abnormalities and osteonecrosis has been well documented with the Gaucher disease. However, most cases of osteonecrosis are associated with simple hypercholesterolemia and/or hypertriglyceridemia. Hyperlipidemia, hyperlipoproteinemia, or abnormally elevated levels of any or all lipids and/or lipoproteins in the blood are other forms of dyslipidemia. It is the most common form of dyslipidemia (which includes any abnormal lipid levels). Hyperlipidemias are divided into primary and secondary subtypes. Primary hyperlipidemia is usually due to genetic causes (such as a mutation in a receptor protein), while secondary hyperlipidemia arises due to other underlying causes such as diabetes. Lipid and lipoprotein abnormalities are common in the general population and are regarded as a modifiable risk factor for cardiovascular disease due to their influence on atherosclerosis. In addition, some forms may predispose to acute pancreatitis. The frequency of familial dyslipidemia varies between 1% and 0.1% according to the type and is much more frequent than osteonecrosis. The rate of osteonecrosis in the general population has been estimated to be between 0.0014% and 0.003%, with the hip being the most common area affected. So even if osteonecrosis is probably a complication of familial dyslipidemia, because osteonecrosis is such a rare complication, its incidence is difficult to accurately analyze. Our case report does not provide conclusive proof that there is a cause–effect relation between dyslipidemia and osteonecrosis. However, the number of patients seen with this condition in our unit has strong presumptive evidence that some association exists and should be researched.

Indication of Hip Arthroplasty in Young Patients

In 1961, Charnley introduced low-friction arthroplasty as an operation suitable for managing older patients and patients with rheumatoid arthritis. More specifically, THA was reserved for patients older than 65 and for patients with severe pain and gross disability. Although Charnley occasionally performed the procedure in middle-aged patients, he did so reluctantly because of concerns regarding long-term survival in younger, more active patients. Historically, several authors described failure rates for THA in osteonecrosis as high as 39–53% with first-generation hip arthroplasty. As results, many authors from 1980 to 1990 have advocated using an osteotomy as an alternative to THA in osteonecrosis, but osteonecrosis volume is often too extensive for osteotomy.

Ultimately, advanced osteonecrosis and failure of the other aggressive interventions mentioned above may necessitate total hip arthroplasty. THA is the most commonly performed procedure for Ficat and ARCO stage III and IV (Steinberg stage IV–VI) osteonecrosis and is highly successful for symptomatic improvement; the durability of THA, however, is inferior to the same procedure performed for osteoarthritis, as patients with osteonecrosis are generally younger and have higher functional demands.

Total hip arthroplasty (THA), an effective treatment for patients with end-stage osteonecrotic hip conditions, provides dramatic pain relief, enhances mobility, and restores function. In every country the demand for THA has risen, and the percentage being performed on patients younger than 30 is increasing steadily and is estimated to be around 10% of the number of arthroplasties.

Is Cemented Arthroplasty an Inconvenience in Young Patients?

The success of THA in older patients, in concert with improvements in techniques and biomaterials, has stimulated demand for this procedure in younger, more active patients hoping to regain full activity. Although young age remains a relative contraindication to THA, the weight of this factor has diminished since 1972, when Charnley reported his first series of patients, whose mean age was less than 65 years. Several investigators have reported cemented THA results in young patients. In patients 18–25 years old, overall implant survival rates have ranged from 65% to 78%, femoral component survival rates from 81% to 95%, and acetabular component survival rates from 68% to 84%. Dorr and colleagues [3] were among the first to analyze the long-term survival of cemented prostheses as related to age and underlying disease, osteoarthritis, rheumatoid arthritis, and avascular necrosis. In a more comprehensive, long-term study, Berry and colleagues [1] compared 25-year survival rates of 2000

THAs performed between 1960 and 1971. Implant survival was strongly associated with patient age and diagnosis at time of procedure. Survival rates decreased with each decade of age.

With improvements being made in cementing and other surgical techniques, the ability to achieve long-term fixation has been enhanced. Younger patient age, however, has been associated with more rapid wear, and accelerated polyethylene wear caused by higher levels of activity and strain on the prosthesis may play a significant role in socket loosening. Ceramic on ceramic may be an option in long-term survival of THAs, because its use has been associated with decreased wear and osteolysis.

Is the Cause of Osteonecrosis a Poor Predictor of Arthroplasty Outcome?

Patients with osteonecrosis are often grouped by associated diseases which can be a risk factor as corticosteroid use, excessive alcohol consumption, and smoking. Recently, organ transplantation (heart, liver, and kidney transplants) and human immunodeficiency virus infection have been found to be associated with osteonecrosis. Some of these diseases might be a cause of worse outcome for THA, and a few studies have reported, for example, increased failure rates in patients with sickle cell disease. The disease disorder may be associated with altered bone remodeling, which may adversely influence fixation of the implant. In some patients, the necrotic lesion may extend into the calcar, with the resultant dead bone providing inadequate support to prevent loosening of the femoral component. Therefore, although osteonecrosis by itself is not an inherent predictor of less favorable outcomes for primary total hip arthroplasty, certain risk factors are associated with higher or lower revision rates [2, 4–21]. However, many patients with osteonecrosis did not have any of these diagnoses, suggesting no poorer outcomes after total hip arthroplasty.

Clinical Pearls and Pitfalls

- Our case report does not provide conclusive proof that there is a cause–effect relation between dyslipidemia and osteonecrosis.
- Total hip arthroplasty (THA), an effective treatment for patients with end-stage osteonecrotic hip conditions, provides dramatic pain relief, enhances mobility, and restores function.
- With improvements being made in cementing and other surgical techniques, cemented THA is a good alternative in the young patient.
- Ceramic on ceramic may be an option in long-term survival of THAs, because its use has been associated with decreased wear and osteolysis.
- Although osteonecrosis by itself is not an inherent predictor of less favorable outcomes for primary total hip arthroplasty, certain risk factors are associated with higher or lower revision rates.

References

1. Barrack RL, Mulroy Jr RD, Harris WH. Improved cementing techniques and femoral component loosening in young patients with hip arthroplasty. A 12-year radiographic review. J Bone Jt Surg Br. 1992;74:385–9.
2. Chiu KY, Ng TP, Tang WM, Poon KC, Ho WY, Yip D. Charnley total hip arthroplasty in Chinese patients less than 40 years old. J Arthroplast. 2001;16:92–101.
3. Dorr LD, Takei GK, Conaty JP. Total hip arthroplasties in patients less than forty-five years old. J Bone Jt Surg Am. 1983;65:474–9.
4. Dudkiewicz I, Covo A, Salai M, Israeli A, Amit Y, Chechik A. Total hip arthroplasty after avascular necrosis of the femoral head: does etiology affect the results? Arch Orthop Trauma Surg. 2004;124:82–5.

5. Goffin E, Baertz G, Rombouts JJ. Long-term survivorship analysis of cemented total hip replacement (THR) after avascular necrosis of the femoral head in renal transplant recipients. Nephrol Dial Transplant. 2006;21:784–8.

6. Ince A, Lermann J, Gobel S, Wollmerstedt N, Hendrich C. No increased stem subsidence after arthroplasty in young patients with femoral head osteonecrosis: 41 patients followed for 1–9 years. Acta Orthop. 2006;77:866–70.

7. Kawasaki M, Hasegawa Y, Sakano S, Masui T, Ishiguro N. Total hip arthroplasty after failed transtrochanteric rotational osteotomy for avascular necrosis of the femoral head. J Arthroplast. 2005;20:574–9.

8. Kim YH, Oh SH, Kim JS, Koo KH. Contemporary total hip arthroplasty with and without cement in patients with osteonecrosis of the femoral head. J Bone Jt Surg Am. 2003;85:675–81.

9. Lebel E, Itzchaki M, Hadas-Halpern I, Zimran A, Elstein D. Outcome of total hip arthroplasty in patients with Gaucher disease. J Arthroplast. 2001;16:7–12.

10. Lieberman JR, Scaduto AA, Wellmeyer E. Symptomatic osteonecrosis of the hip after orthotopic liver transplantation. J Arthroplast. 2000;15:767–71.

11. Moran MC, Huo MH, Garvin KL, Pellicci PM, Salvati EA. Total hip arthroplasty in sickle cell hemoglobinopathy. Clin Orthop Relat Res. 1993;294:140–8.

12. Nich C, Courpied JP, Kerboull M, Postel M, Hamadouche M. Charnley-Kerboull total hip arthroplasty for osteonecrosis of the femoral head a minimal 10-year follow-up study. J Arthroplast. 2006;21:533–40.

13. Nich C, Sariali el H, Hannouche D, Nizard R, Witvoet J, Sedel L, Bizot P. Long-term results of alumina-on-alumina hip arthroplasty for osteonecrosis. Clin Orthop Relat Res. 2003;417:102–11.

14. Ritter MA, Helphinstine J, Keating EM, Faris PM, Meding JB. Total hip arthroplasty in patients with osteonecrosis. The effect of cement techniques. Clin Orthop Relat Res. 1997;338:94–9.

15. Saito S, Saito M, Nishina T, Ohzono K, Ono K. Long-term results of total hip arthroplasty for osteonecrosis of the femoral head. A comparison with osteoarthritis. Clin Orthop Relat Res. 1989;244:198–207.

16. Schneider W, Knahr K. Total hip replacement in younger patients: survival rate after avascular necrosis of the femoral head. Acta Orthop Scand. 2004;75:142–6.

17. Seyler TM, Bonutti PM, Shen J, Naughton M, Kester M. Use of an alumina-on-alumina bearing system in total hip arthroplasty for osteonecrosis of the hip. J Bone Jt Surg Am. 2006;88(Suppl 3):116–25.
18. Steinberg ME, Lai M, Garino JP, Ong A, Wong KL. A comparison between total hip replacement for osteonecrosis and degenerative joint disease. Orthopedics. 2008;31:360.
19. Wroblewski BM, Siney PD, Fleming PA. Charnley low-frictional torque arthroplasty for avascular necrosis of the femoral head. J Arthroplast. 2005;20:870–3. doi:10.1016/j.arth.2005.02.006.
20. Xenakis TA, Beris AE, Malizos KK, Koukoubis T, Gelalis J, Soucacos PN. Total hip arthroplasty for avascular necrosis and degenerative osteoarthritis of the hip. Clin Orthop Relat Res. 1997;341:62–8.
21. Zangger P, Gladman DD, Urowitz MB, Bogoch ER. Outcome of total hip replacement for avascular necrosis in systemic lupus erythematosus. J Rheumatol. 2000;27:919–23.

Chapter 21
Complications of Uncemented Total Hip Arthroplasty: Success

Carlos J. Lavernia, Michele D'Apuzzo, and Jesus M. Villa

Case Presentation

A 36-year-old female Hispanic patient, with history of pituitary adenoma requiring removal in April of 1993 with subsequent use of dexamethasone, presented for the first time to the office in May 1994 complaining of severe bilateral hip pain. The pain was intermittent at night and it was partially relieved by Naproxen. There was no limitation in her walk-

C.J. Lavernia, MD (✉)
Voluntary Professor, University of Miami,
Florida International University, 2550 SW 37th Avenue #301,
Coral Gables, FL 33134, USA
e-mail: c@drlavernia.com

M. D'Apuzzo, MD
The Center for Advanced Orthopaedics at Larkin,
7000 SW 62nd Ave, Suite 600, South Miami, FL 33143, USA
e-mail: mdapuzzo@larkinhospital.com

J.M. Villa, MD
Arthritis Surgery Research Foundation,
2550 SW 37th Avenue #301, Coral Gables, FL 33134, USA
e-mail: jesus@drlavernia.net

R.J. Sierra (ed.), *Osteonecrosis of the Femoral Head*,
DOI 10.1007/978-3-319-50664-7_21,
© Mayo Foundation for Medical Education and Research 2017

ing distance and no need of any assistive device. At physical examination, the patient had a mildly antalgic gait and leg length was equal. Hip range of motion was symmetrical on both sides and consisted of flexion 110°, internal rotation 40°, external rotation 30°, abduction 20°, and adduction 40°.

Diagnosis/Assessment

The patient brought radiographs which demonstrated bilateral osteonecrosis of the femoral heads without collapse. The lesions, in both hips, were classified according to the staging system of Steinberg et al. [1] as stage IIB (cystic and sclerotic changes in the femoral head with 15–30% of femoral head compromise). [2] (Figs. 21.1 and 21.2).

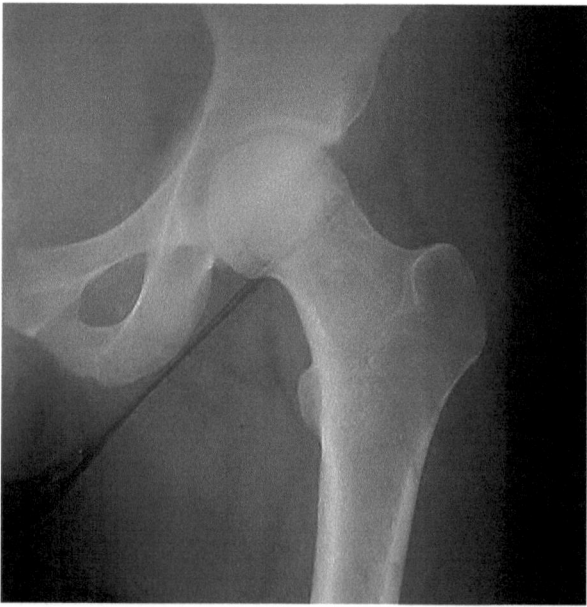

FIGURE 21.1 Anteroposterior radiograph of the left hip before the core decompression. There is good articular space and no evidence of collapse of the femoral head

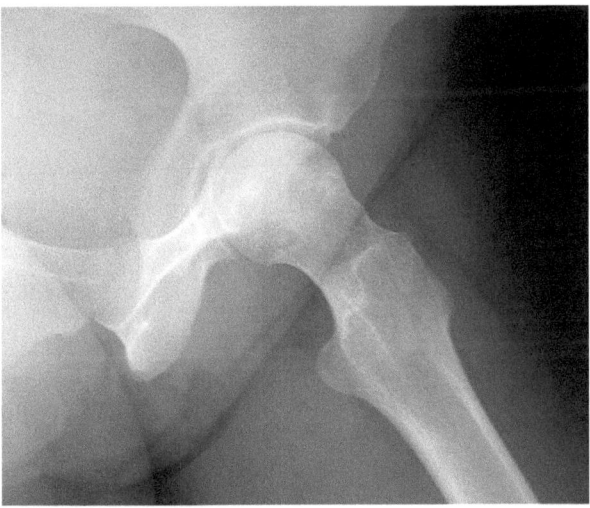

FIGURE 21.2 Lateral radiograph of the left hip before the core decompression. There is good articular space and no indication of femoral head collapse

Management

The patient underwent bilateral core decompression in June 1994. An 11 mm drill was inserted in to the lesion under fluoroscopy, followed by partial coring of the lesion with a curette which was then taken through the same incision. Postoperatively, the patient was wheelchair bound and allowed only bathroom transfers for 6 weeks with advanced weight bearing over the following 4 weeks. Pathology confirmed the diagnosis of osteonecrosis in both femoral heads.

Outcome Bilateral Core Decompression

The patient recovered from both procedures uneventfully. At 3 months postoperatively, she complained only of slight pain in the right hip while the left hip was pain free. Thereafter, she started full weight bearing as tolerated. Approximately 5 months

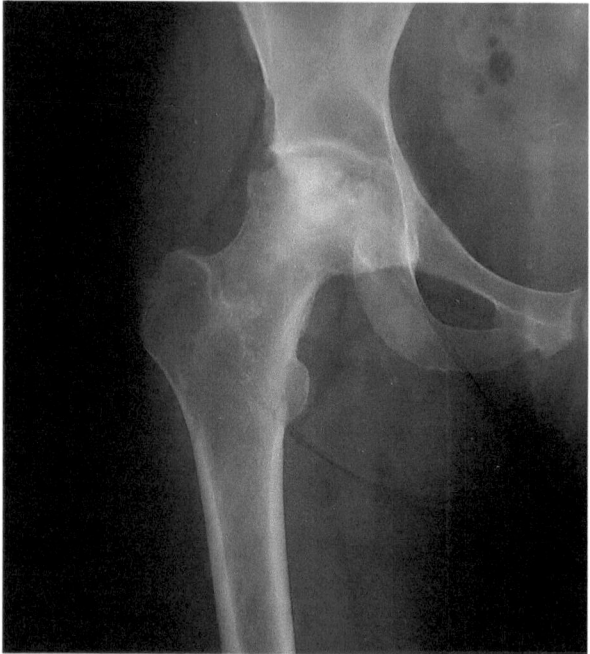

FIGURE 21.3 Anteroposterior radiograph of the right hip after the core decompression demonstrating collapse of the femoral head and a subchondral fracture

after the procedures, she started dancing and complained thereafter of severe pain in the right hip. The patient was promptly evaluated and found to have collapse with subchondral fracture of the femoral head in the right hip (Fig. 21.3).

She was placed on crutches with significant improvement of her pain, to the point that after 2 weeks they pain resolved. Then, weight bearing was restarted as tolerated up to full weight bearing. For several years, the patient complained only intermittently from pain in the right hip (moderate at most) but overall she did well and lived a completely normal life; including dancing. Nine years after the core decompressions, she remained pain free with a normal gait and flexion of 120° in both hips. Internal rotation on the right side was 10° and 40°

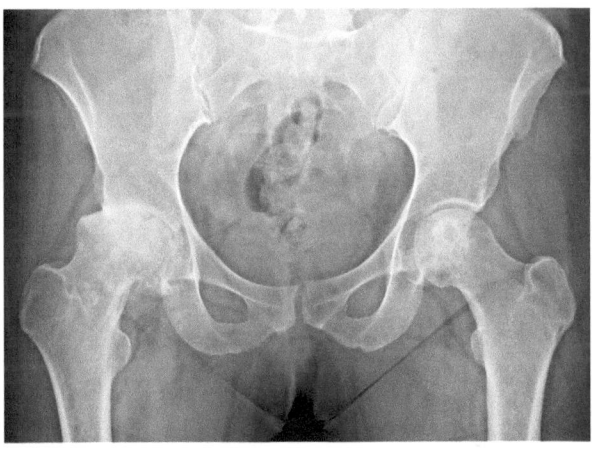

Figure 21.4 Anteroposterior radiograph of the pelvis demonstrating collapse of the femoral head and arthrosis of the right hip 20 years after the core decompression. The left hip shows no signs of collapse, and it also shows good preservation of the articular space (20 years after the core decompression)

on the left side. Thirteen years after both procedures, the patient was happy with the results and only had mild periodic pain without need for pain medications. Twenty years after the bilateral core decompression, in 2014, the patient complained of pain in the right hip; this pain was progressively worse for the last 6 years. The pain in the right hip was worsened by standing and by long periods of activity, and it was improved by walking. There were no flexion contractures bilaterally. Flexion was 90° on the right side and 100° on the left, internal rotation was 0° (right) and 35° (left), external rotation was 30° (right) and 45° (left), abduction was 20° (right) and 45° (left), and adduction was 10° on the right side and 45° on the left hip. The right hip radiographs demonstrated complete collapse of the femoral head, joint space was bone on bone, subchondral sclerosis on both the femur and acetabular side, and clear femoral head deformity from previous collapse (Figs. 21.4 and 21.5). The patient decided 20 years after the core decompression to finally undergo a right total hip arthroplasty.

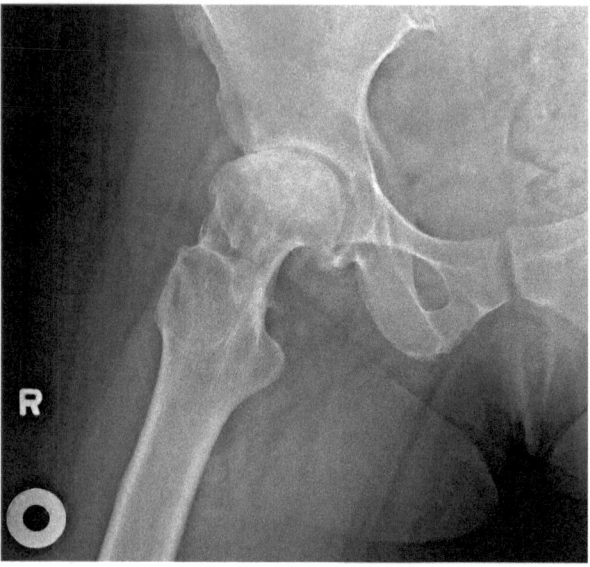

FIGURE 21.5 Lateral radiograph of the right hip demonstrating loss of articular space 20 years after the core decompression

Outcome

Postoperatively, the patient evolved uneventfully. Six months after surgery, she was able to walk without limitations and to go up the stairs normally holding to the rail. She is currently satisfied with the surgery and performs her routine daily life activities successfully and without any limitations (Figs. 21.6 and 21.7).

Literature Review

This case illustrates how the exposure to steroids is indeed an important factor in the development of osteonecrosis of the femoral head. It also demonstrates how the preservation of the femoral head thanks to a core decompression may be

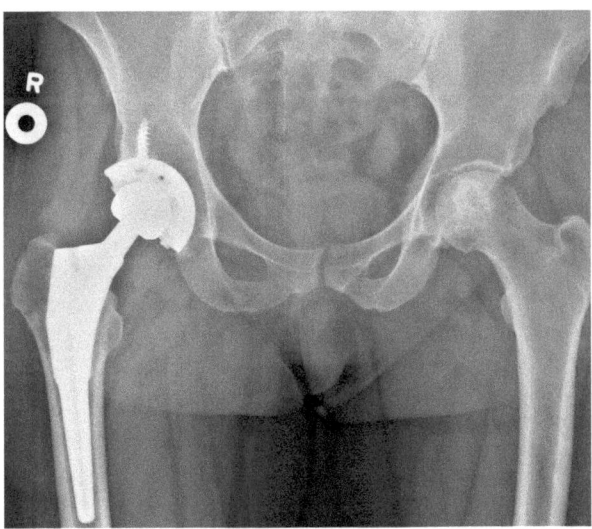

FIGURE 21.6 Anteroposterior radiograph of the pelvis performed after cementless right total hip arthroplasty

attempted in younger patients without head collapse [3]. The left side in this case still remains pain free 21 years after the core decompression. In the early stages, the first radiographic findings usually consist of cystic and sclerotic changes in the femoral head as clearly demonstrated in this patient [4, 5]. One of the lessons that we can draw from this particular case is that, due to the low risk, core decompression should be attempted to prevent the collapse of the femoral head. This is particularly important in younger patients. In this particular case, it allowed the patient to receive a better articulating surface since most of the polyethylene used in 1993 was not highly cross-linked and for sure would have required at least one revision in the last 20 years.

This case also shows that even in face of femoral head collapse, total hip arthroplasty reliably achieves rapid pain relief and functional recovery with a single procedure. Recent series with longer follow-up regarding the use of cementless THA for osteonecrosis are encouraging, with reported

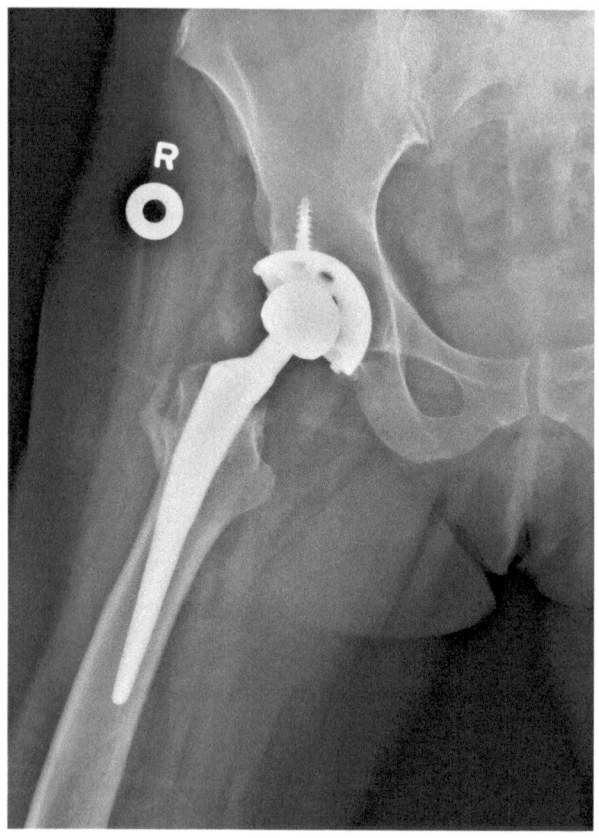

FIGURE 21.7 Lateral radiograph of the right hip performed after total hip arthroplasty

long-term survivorships exceeding 90%. Kim et al. [6], using modular stem cementless THAs in patients younger than 50 years, reported 93.8% of survivorship at a minimum follow-up of 15 years using stem revision for any reason as the end point (for aseptic loosening exclusively, the survivorship was 100%). As noted by the group of Callaghan, [7] the long-term survivorship of cementless THAs in patients with osteonecrosis encourages us to continue to use cementless devices in these patients. Michael Mont and his group reported a 95% aseptic implant survivorship at a mean follow-up of approximately 7.5 years in patients diagnosed with sickle cell disease. [8] It cannot be overemphasized that early diagnosis and treatment with core decompression are crucial to preserve the femoral head, but in face of collapse, a cementless THA consistently achieves immediate pain relief and functional recovery. Johnson et al. [9] performed a 16-year analysis of the Nationwide Inpatient Sample concerning the treatment of femoral head osteonecrosis in the United States. The report suggests an improvement in the survivorship of THA since 1993. In 1992, 75% of the procedures performed to treat hip osteonecrosis were total hip arthroplasty, but this figure increased to 88% in 2008. During the same period of time, the rate of joint-preserving procedures dropped from 25% to 12%. Surgeons are more frequently performing total hip arthroplasty to treat patients with osteonecrosis, and as a result, an increasing percentage of osteonecrosis patients are currently treated with THA.

In summary, and in spite of the variety of procedures proposed to treat this particular condition [10–12], a simple core decompression in face of pre-collapse lesions and a total hip arthroplasty in presence of collapse and/or arthrosis of the femoral head appear to be dependable and recognized options for the treatment of osteonecrosis of the femoral head.

Clinical Pearls and Pitfalls

- Core decompression should always be considered in young patients with osteonecrosis of the femoral head without collapse. This is of utmost importance in younger patients.
- Currently, total hip arthroplasty is associated with excellent survivorship in those cases with diagnosis of osteonecrosis of the femoral head

References

1. Steinberg ME, Hayken GD, Steinberg DR. A quantitative system for staging avascular necrosis. J Bone Joint Surg (Br). 1995;77(1):34–41.
2. Lavernia CJ, Sierra RJ, Grieco FR. Osteonecrosis of the femoral head. J Am Acad Orthop Surg. 1999;7(4):250–61.
3. Lavernia CJ, Sierra RJ. Core decompression in atraumatic osteonecrosis of the hip. J Arthroplast. 2000;15(2):171–8.
4. Zalavras CG, Lieberman JR. Osteonecrosis of the femoral head: evaluation and treatment. J Am Acad Orthop Surg. 2014; 22(7):455–64.
5. Lieberman JR, Engstrom SM, Meneghini RM, SooHoo NF. Which factors influence preservation of the osteonecrotic femoral head? Clin Orthop Relat Res. 2012;470(2):525–34.
6. Kim SM, Lim SJ, Moon YW, Kim YT, Ko KR, Park YS. Cementless modular total hip arthroplasty in patients younger than fifty with femoral head osteonecrosis: minimum fifteen-year follow-up. J Arthroplast. 2013;28(3):504–9.
7. Bedard NA, Callaghan JJ, Liu SS, Greiner JJ, Klaassen AL, Johnston RC. Cementless THA for the treatment of osteonecrosis at 10-year follow-up: have we improved compared to cemented THA? J Arthroplast. 2013;28(7):1192–9.
8. Issa K, Naziri Q, Maheshwari AV, Rasquinha VJ, Delanois RE, Mont MA. Excellent results and minimal complications of total hip arthroplasty in sickle cell hemoglobinopathy at mid-term follow-up using cementless prosthetic components. J Arthroplast. 2013;28(9):1693–8.
9. Johnson AJ, Mont MA, Tsao AK, Jones LC. Treatment of femoral head osteonecrosis in the United States: 16-year analysis of the Nationwide Inpatient Sample. Clin Orthop Relat Res. 2014;472(2):617–23.
10. Sen RK, Tripathy SK, Aggarwal S, Marwaha N, Sharma RR, Khandelwal N. Early results of core decompression and autologous bone marrow mononuclear cells instillation in femoral head osteonecrosis: a randomized control study. J Arthroplast. 2012;27(5):679–86.

11. Cui Q, Botchwey EA. Emerging ideas: treatment of precollapse osteonecrosis using stem cells and growth factors. Clin Orthop Relat Res. 2011;469(9):2665–9.
12. Papanagiotou M, Malizos KN, Vlychou M, Dailiana ZH. Autologous (non-vascularised) fibular grafting with recombinant bone morphogenetic protein-7 for the treatment of femoral head osteonecrosis: preliminary report. Bone Joint J. 2014;96-B(1):31–5.

Chapter 22
Complications of Uncemented Total Hip Arthroplasty: Failure

Michele D'Apuzzo, Carlos J. Lavernia, and Jesus M. Villa

Case Presentation

A 56-year-old white male patient presented to the office with a history of constant pain in both hips. In both cases, pain was graded in intensity and frequency as eight and ten points, respectively [visual analogue scale (VAS); range, 0–10]. The patient was able to walk between two and five blocks, and he had to use a crutch

---

M. D'Apuzzo, MD
The Center for Advanced Orthopaedics at Larkin,
7000 SW 62nd Ave, Suite 600, South Miami, FL 33143, USA
e-mail: mdapuzzo@larkinhospital.com

C.J. Lavernia, MD (✉)
Voluntary Professor, University of Miami,
Florida International University, 2550 SW 37th Avenue #301,
Coral Gables, FL 33134, USA
e-mail: c@drlavernia.com

J.M. Villa, MD
Arthritis Surgery Research Foundation,
2550 SW 37th Avenue #301, Coral Gables, FL 33134, USA
e-mail: jesus@drlavernia.net

R.J. Sierra (ed.), *Osteonecrosis of the Femoral Head*,
DOI 10.1007/978-3-319-50664-7_22,
© Mayo Foundation for Medical Education and Research 2017

all of the time. He was able to go upstairs or downstairs only one step at a time. Both hips were treated with total hip arthroplasty which were performed under the same anesthesia. On the right side, the whole postoperative period was uneventful and had excellent outcomes up to the latest follow-up. Unfortunately, the story of the left THA was quite different. Preoperatively, flexion in the left hip was 70°, abduction/adduction was 30°, internal rotation was 0°, and external rotation was 10°. For the purposes of this illustrative case-based chapter, we will focus on the left hip.

Diagnosis/Assessment

The anteroposterior radiographs of the left hip demonstrated complete obliteration of the hip articular space as well as secondary osteoarthrosis of both the femur and the acetabulum with associated collapse of the femoral head. The lateral view showed similar findings. The patient was diagnosed with osteonecrosis of the femoral head. (Figs. 22.1 and 22.2)

Management

Due to pain and functional limitations, the patient underwent a cementless left total hip arthroplasty using a tapered stem. (Figs. 22.3 and 22.4). Postoperatively, the patient had no restrictions on weight bearing, and he was discharged from the hospital without incidents.

Outcome

The immediate postoperative period went uneventfully. At 6 months of follow-up, the patient had no pain and his walking distance was unlimited. The Harris Hip Score at this point

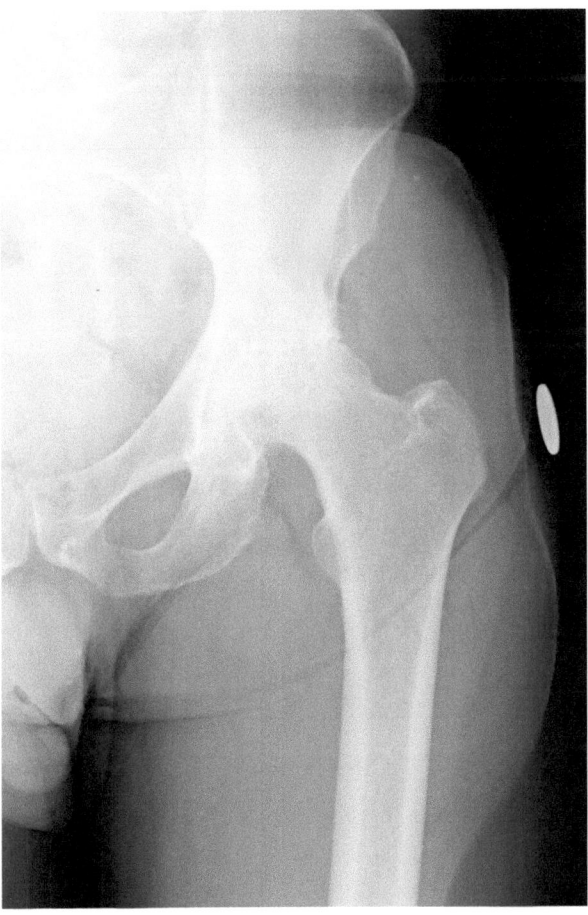

FIGURE 22.1 Anteroposterior radiograph of the left hip demonstrating loss of articular space and flattening of the femoral head

in time was 100 points. At about 2 years after surgery, however, the patient complained of anterior pain in the upper thigh in what appeared to be a strain of the sartorius or the rectus femoris, and he was placed on anti-inflammatory medication. Soon thereafter, the pain increased in

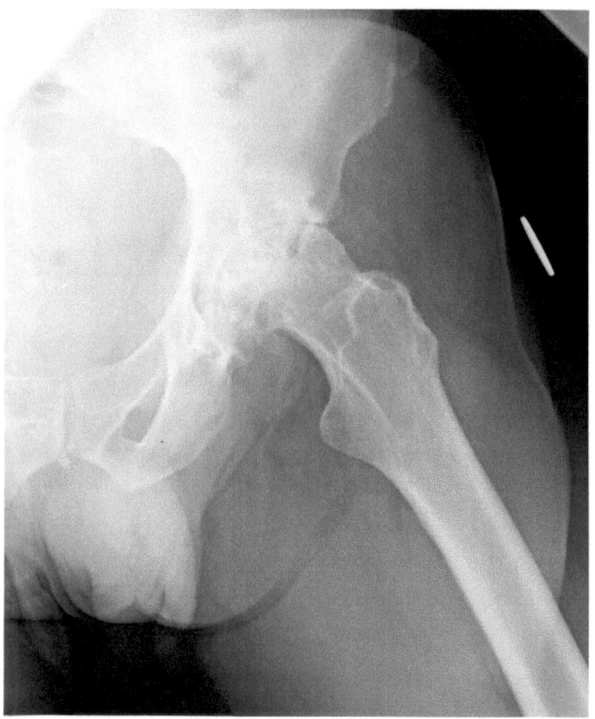

FIGURE 22.2 Lateral radiograph of the left hip showing minimal joint space and flattening of the femoral head

intensity and frequency to ten points (VAS), and the walking distance of the patient decreased to one block. He had to use a cane at all times. Consequently, an aspiration and arthrocentesis was performed on the left hip, and the culture result was positive: *staphylococcus aureus* was isolated. The preoperative radiograph at this moment is shown in Fig. 22.5. With a diagnosis of deep infection, intravenous cefazolin was started via a Groshong catheter for a period of 6 weeks, and the patient was scheduled for resection of the hip prosthesis and insertion of an antibiotic cement spacer (Fig. 22.6). A few days after surgery, unfortunately, the spacer dislocated (Figs. 22.7) and it was removed (Figs. 22.8 and 22.9). Three

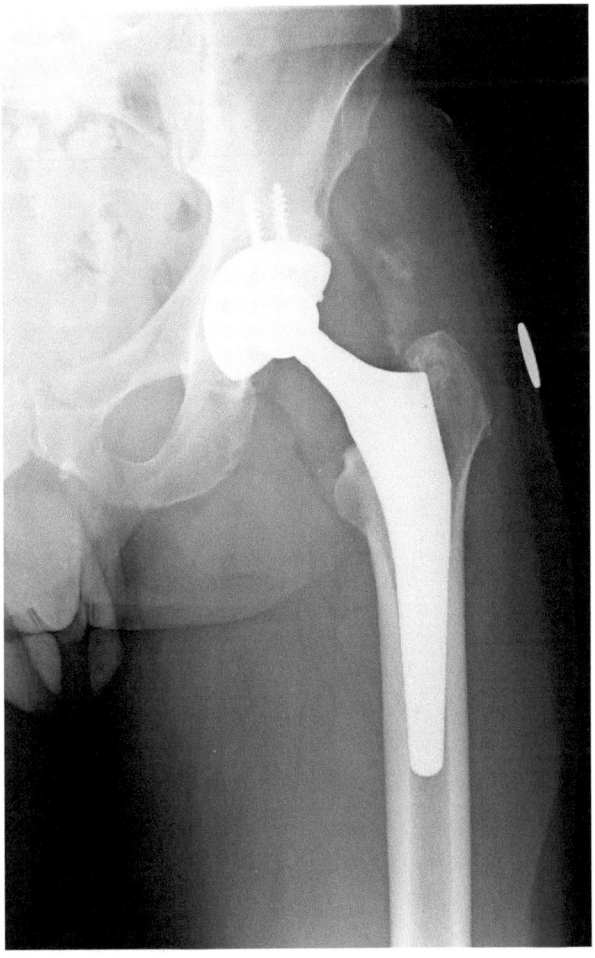

FIGURE 22.3 Anteroposterior radiograph of the left hip taken approximately 3 months after cementless total hip arthroplasty

months later, an open biopsy was performed and the cultures obtained were negative. Approximately 2 months after this, the patient underwent a left THA reimplantation (Figs. 22.10 and 22.11). The immediate postoperative period proceeded without incident, and the patient was delighted with the

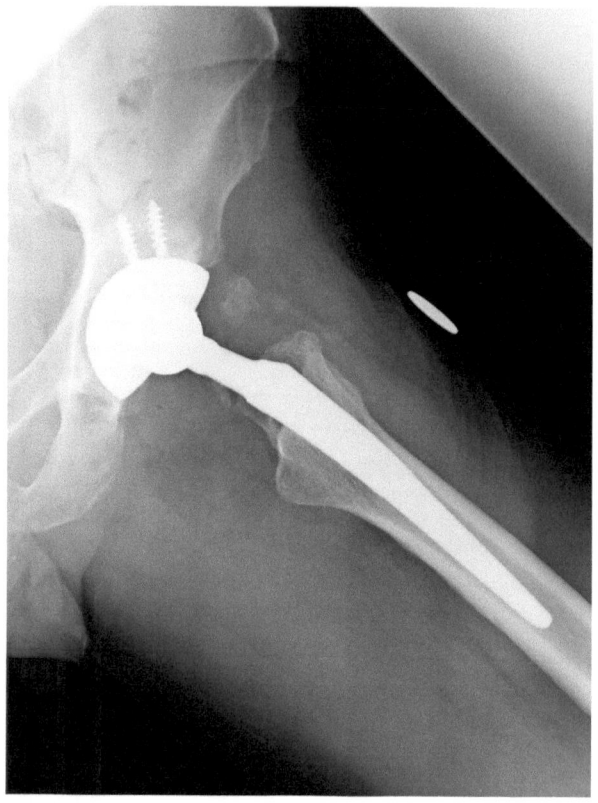

FIGURE 22.4 Lateral radiograph of the left hip obtained approximately 3 months after cementless total hip arthroplasty

results without complaints. Two years after the reimplantation, there was no pain and the walking distance was unlimited. The Harris Hip Score was 95 and the patient was satisfied with the procedure.

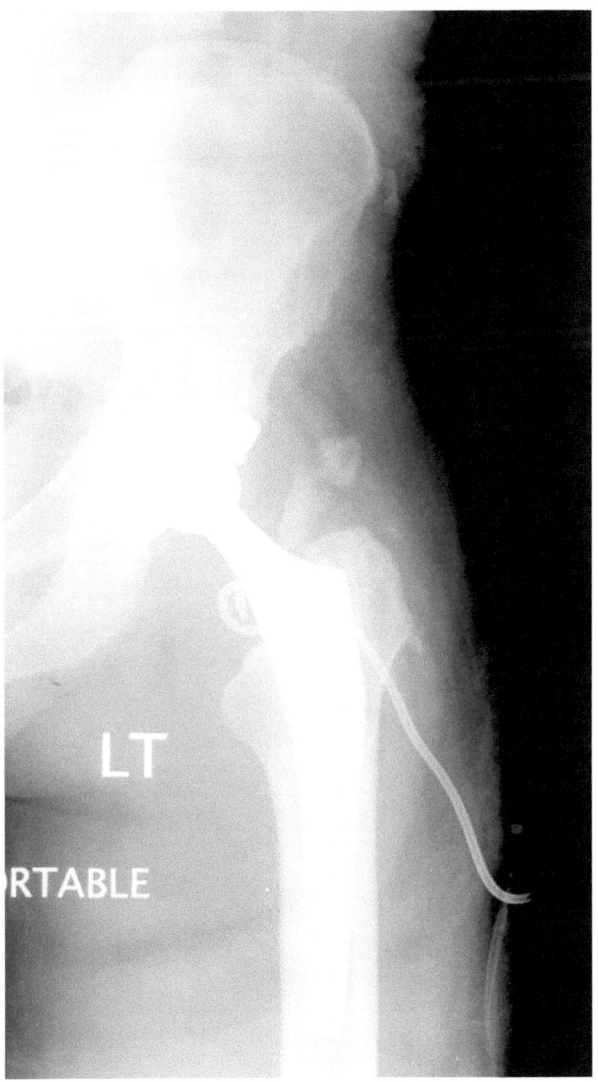

FIGURE 22.5 Anteroposterior radiograph of the left hip obtained before implant removal

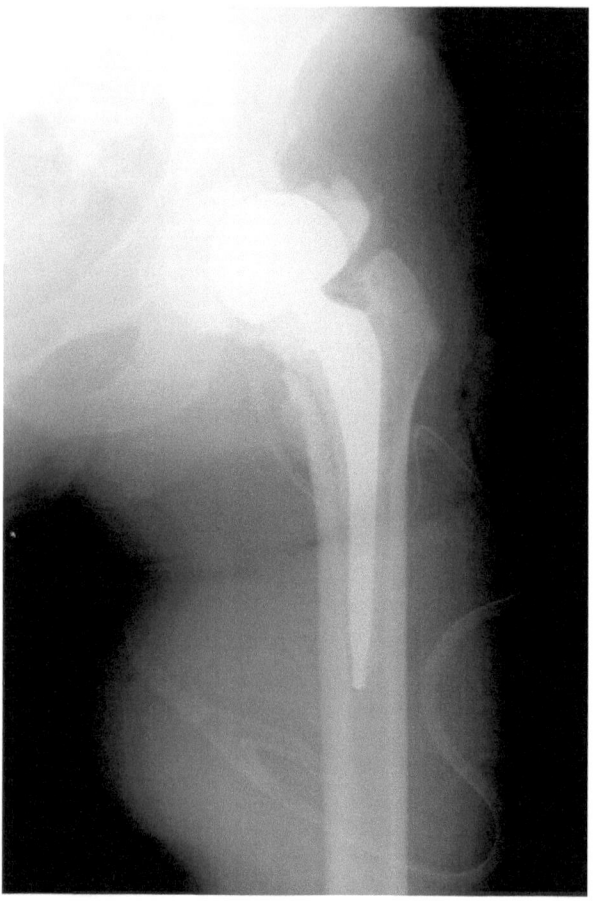

FIGURE 22.6 Anteroposterior radiograph of the left hip showing articulating spacer in place

Literature Review

Contemporary series [1, 2] have demonstrated excellent results obtained with the use of total hip arthroplasty when performed for femoral head osteonecrosis. The general

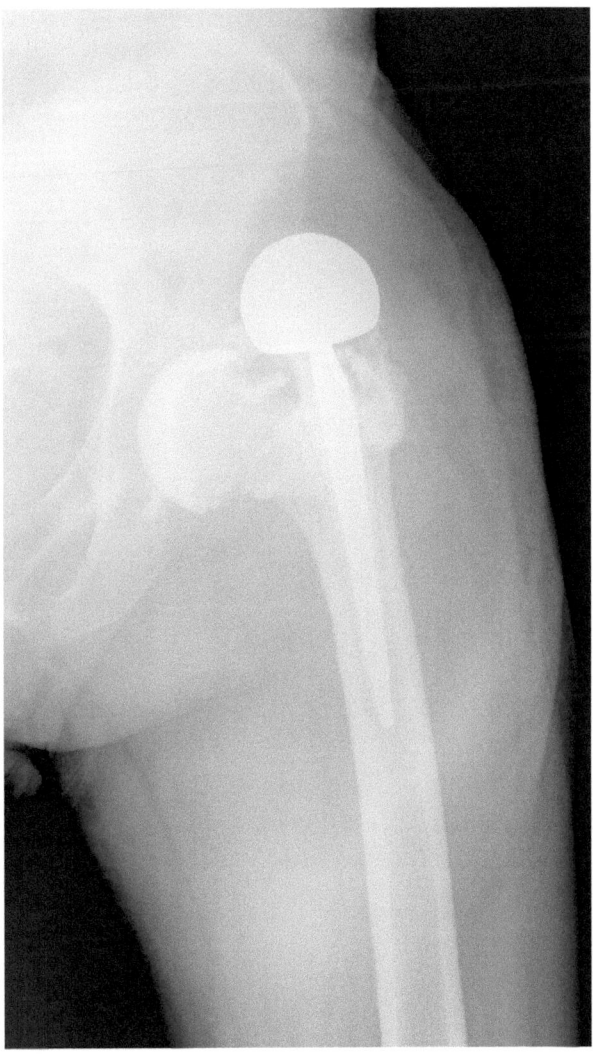

FIGURE 22.7 Anteroposterior radiograph of the left hip demonstrating dislocation of the spacer

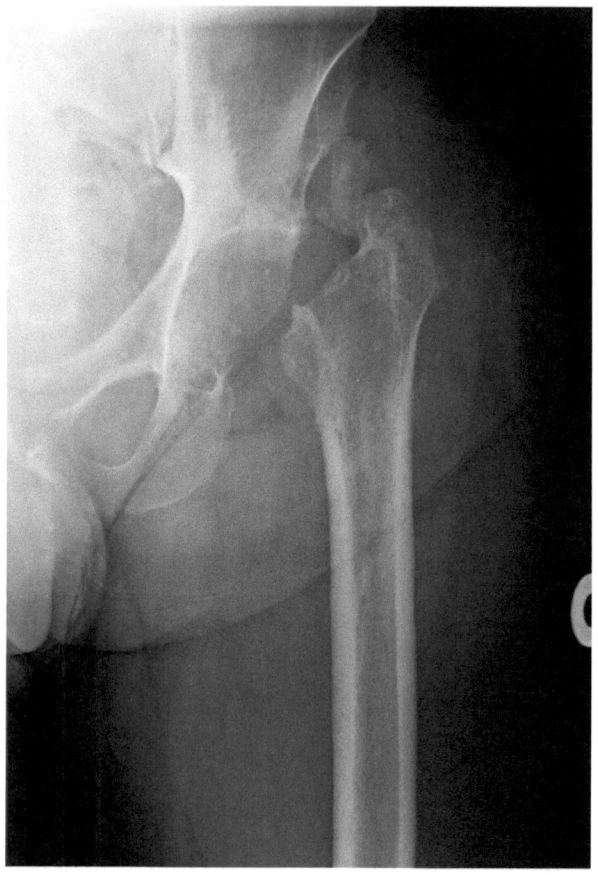

FIGURE 22.8 Anteroposterior radiograph of the left hip after removal of the spacer

association of poor outcomes with THA performed in patients with this diagnosis belongs to the past. Nevertheless, the results of the arthroplasty are still dependent on the original disease responsible for the osteonecrosis of the femoral head. The deep infection case illustrated here might as well occur with a primary THA performed for any other diagnosis, but this particular complication should always be considered

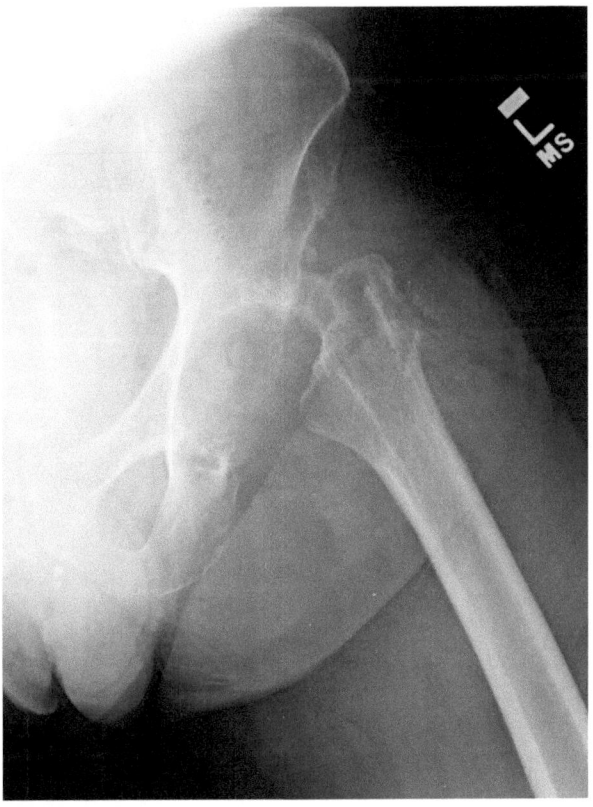

FIGURE 22.9 Lateral radiograph of the left hip after spacer removal

in those cases performed in patients with osteonecrosis associated with sickle cell disease or immunologic conditions although excellent results can still be achieved in these. Woo et al. [3] studied a series of 19 THAs performed in 13 patients diagnosed with osteonecrosis and systemic lupus erythematosus (SLE). The results of these cases where compared with a control group of patients with osteonecrosis but without SLE. The authors found no significant differences in the Harris Hip Scores between both groups. Further, there were no infections or any other significant complication related to

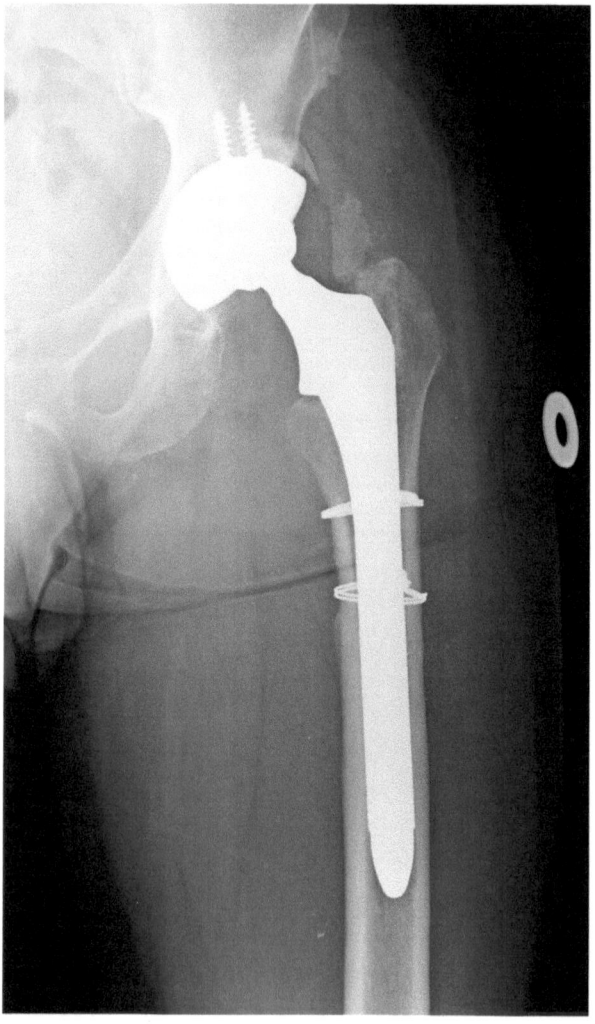

Figure 22.10 Anteroposterior radiograph of the left hip obtained after reimplantation of the total hip arthroplasty

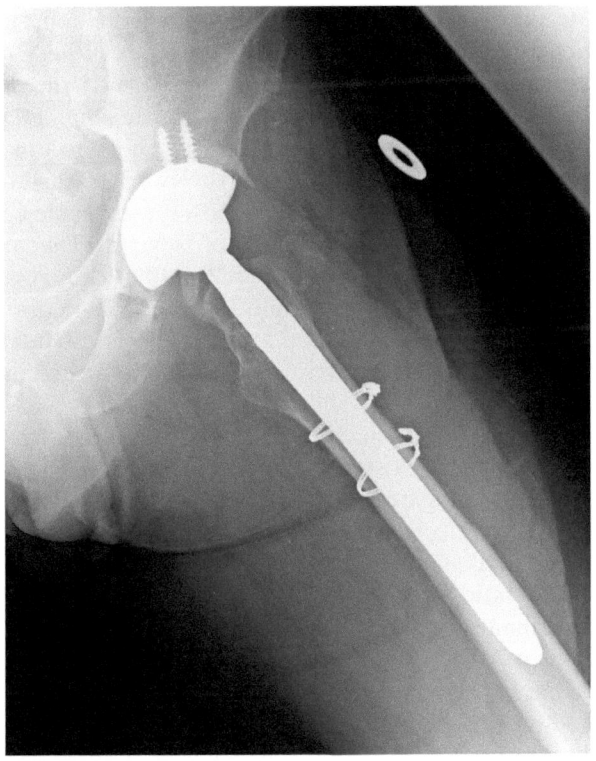

FIGURE 22.11 Lateral radiograph of the reimplantation of the left total hip arthroplasty

the surgery. Issa et al. [4] compared 32 sickle cell patients (42 hips) with 87 non-sickle cell osteonecrosis patients (102 hips) and found that there were no significant differences in aseptic prosthesis survivorship, Harris Hip scores, SF-36, or on radiographic findings. There was no deep infection in the non-sickle cell osteonecrosis group, but in the sickle cell cohort, two patients were revised due to septic loosening at about 6 months and 13 months after the index surgery. A two-stage exchange revision surgery was performed successfully in both cases, and a Harris Hip Score greater than 80 points was achieved after the reimplantation (similar to our case). Hernigou et al. [5] retrospectively reviewed 312 arthroplasties performed in 244 patients diagnosed with sickle cell disease with a minimum follow-up of 5 years. The authors observed a rate of late infection of 3% (10/312). A two-stage exchange revision was performed for infection 45 days after removal of the initial arthroplasty. At the latest follow-up, eight of the ten hips had no infection but two had recurrence of it.

In summary, complications due to infection seem to be more prevalent in those patients diagnosed with osteonecrosis and immunologic conditions and/or sickle cell disease. The rates of deep infection are particularly concerning. However, due to the excellent results achieved in some series, the risk-to-benefit ratio seems to be reasonable and total hip arthroplasty remains a valid option even for these patients.

Sickle cell disease patients undergoing THA need a special and complex perioperative workup. Patients should have a complete hematologic evaluation including antibody screening before surgery. All blood products should be typed for ABO, Rhesus, and Kell to prevent antigen mismatch during transfusions. Red blood cell exchange (aimed to decrease hemoglobin S level to less than 30%) should be considered in those patients with a history of acute chest syndrome, cerebrovascular episode, or severe anemia (<5 g/dL). To decrease the risk of infection, patients with gallstones should have their gallbladder removed before surgery. If cement were to be used, it should contain antibiotics. In addition, antibiotic prophylaxis should be extended for 3 days after surgery [5]. In order to decrease the risk of clotting in small vessels, all patients with sickle cell disease undergoing THA should be admitted the night before surgery and have IV hydration started at midnight.

Clinical Pearls and Pitfalls

- Overall, the results of current THA for osteonecrosis are excellent. However, these results are still dependent on the original disease responsible for the osteonecrosis of the femoral head.
- Deep infection remains a concern in those cases performed for osteonecrosis with sickle cell disease and/or immunologic conditions. However, the risk-to-benefit ratio seems reasonable and total hip arthroplasty remains a valid option even for these patients.

References

1. Kim SM, Lim SJ, Moon YW, Kim YT, Ko KR, Park YS. Cementless modular total hip arthroplasty in patients younger than fifty with femoral head osteonecrosis: minimum fifteen-year follow-up. J Arthroplast. 2013;28(3):504–9.
2. Bedard NA, Callaghan JJ, Liu SS, Greiner JJ, Klaassen AL, Johnston RC. Cementless THA for the treatment of osteonecrosis at 10-year follow-up: have we improved compared to cemented THA? J Arthroplast. 2013;28(7):1192–9.
3. Woo MS, Kang JS, Moon KH. Outcome of total hip arthroplasty for avascular necrosis of the femoral head in systemic lupus erythematosus. J Arthroplast. 2014;29(12):2267–70.
4. Issa K, Naziri Q, Maheshwari AV, Rasquinha VJ, Delanois RE, Mont MA. Excellent results and minimal complications of total hip arthroplasty in sickle cell hemoglobinopathy at mid-term follow-up using cementless prosthetic components. J Arthroplast. 2013;28(9):1693–8.
5. Hernigou P, Zilber S, Filippini P, Mathieu G, Poignard A, Galacteros F. Total THA in adult osteonecrosis related to sickle cell disease. Clin Orthop Relat Res. 2008;466(2):300–8.

Index

R.J. Sierra (ed.), *Osteonecrosis of the Femoral Head*,
DOI 10.1007/978-3-319-50664-7,
© Mayo Foundation for Medical Education and Research 2017